Clinical Integration

Mary Crabtree Tonges, Editor

Foreword by Karen Zander, RN

Clinical Integration

Strategies and Practices for Organized Delivery Systems

Jossey-Bass Publishers • San Francisco

Jossey-Bass books and products are available through most
bookstores. To contact Jossey-Bass directly, call (888) 378-2537, fax
to (800) 605-2665, or visit our website at www.josseybass.com.

Substantial discounts on bulk quantities of Jossey-Bass books are
available to corporations, professional associations, and other
organizations. For details and discount information, contact the
special sales department at Jossey-Bass.

For sales outside the United States, please contact your local Simon
& Schuster International Office.

 Manufactured in the United States of America on Lyons Falls
Turin Book. This paper is acid-free and 100 percent totally
chlorine-free.

Library of Congress Cataloging-in-Publication Data

Clinical integration : strategies and practices for organized delivery
systems / Mary Tonges, editor.—1st ed.
        p.   cm.
    Includes index.
    ISBN 0-7879-4039-9 (alk. paper)
    1. Integrated delivery of health care.   2. Health services
administration.   I. Tonges, Mary Crabtree.
    [DNLM: 1. Delivery of Health Care, Integrated.   2. Health
Services—organization & administration.   W 84 C641 1998]
RA394.C56   1998
362.1'068—dc21
DNLM/DLC
for Library of Congress   98-2503

FIRST EDITION
HB Printing   10 9 8 7 6 5 4 3 2 1

Contents

Tables and Figures

Foreword

Clinical integration is a fairly new concept more easily defined by its absence or by the confusion it sparks than by any clear understanding. This book is the first to explain clinical integration at the professional level, where it is practiced daily.

Having seen many examples of the lack of consistency, communication, standards, and even common sense in the delivery of health care, every reader will appreciate the challenges of operationalizing integrated delivery. The challenge to any one health care agency to become a perfect whole is staggering, let alone a group of agencies, physicians, and others that are now supposed to perform as a system. Physicians, nurses, and administrators are well aware that their organizations weren't perfect before the economic upheaval of the 1990s; and, while ever hopeful of improvement, they realize that perfection remains a distant goal. A coordinated effort that aspires to clinical integration brings that goal closer.

Clinical Integration outlines clear theories and interpretations that, taken together, represent a fundamental presence of coordinated continuous health care across operating units that service whatever level of care a person's health status requires. The book then moves the reader to practices that have already shown success. Those practices come in the form of tools, roles, and relationships for planning, delivering, managing, and evaluating clinical processes that are provided in the most appropriate venue, with the goal of maximizing measurable health outcomes at the least cost.

Once the value equation of quality and cost is discovered for each major patient population, the health system has to restructure itself to support the equation with a reliable, responsive infrastructure. This book focuses on specific types of infrastructure along with the need for ongoing evaluation of the fit between the current infrastructure and the more fluid value equation.

The scope of clinical integration includes by its nature very detailed work. To quote this book's editor, Mary Crabtree Tonges, all good ideas eventually must regress to the hard work of implementation. Clinical integration is no exception. Health systems must respond to the many challenges raised as they strive to create better integration of patient care services:

- Creating a common language and common culture while preserving pride and autonomy
- Aligning incentives when information is lacking or not trusted
- Keeping clinicians in tune with best practices against an accelerated learning curve
- Developing the competencies managers and administrators need to lead an immensely interdependent set of variables that must produce transactions precisely and humanely, one patient at a time

Clinical Integration begins where other books on similar topics have ended: where theory becomes practice. This book's mission is to assist health care organizations to push aggressively beyond business and contractual relationships, to the task of restructuring clinical processes, content, and philosophy. Your success in taking this knowledge and turning it into action will show that this book has fulfilled its mission.

South Natick, Massachusetts KAREN ZANDER, RN
March 1998

Acknowledgments

To Jim, Christina, and Jack: Mom got the dissertation, and this book's for you, with grateful thanks for your support and accommodations. You make anything good that I do possible.

I also want to thank Karen Zander and Kathleen Bower for the many professional opportunities they've given me, including this one, and the chance to be a part of the Center for Case Management team. I am grateful to my friend and colleague Ann Scott Blouin for suggesting authors and for many other kindnesses.

Next, and very importantly, I offer sincere thanks to each of the contributors to this book, without whose talent and commitment it clearly would not exist. I also thank Andy Pasternack for graciously assisting a first-time editor. Finally the anonymous reviewers' insightful and valuable comments are gratefully acknowledged.

M.C.T.

The Editor

MARY CRABTREE TONGES is senior vice president of nursing and patient services at the Robert Wood Johnson University Hospital (RWJUH), and a national and international consultant with the Center for Case Management. She received her B.S.N. degree (1973) from the University of Iowa, her M.S.N. degree (1977) from the University of Illinois, and her M.B.A. (1995) and Ph.D. (1997) degrees in organization and policy studies from Baruch College of the City University of New York.

Tonges has held clinical faculty appointments in nursing administration at the University of Illinois, Northwestern University, and Rutgers Colleges of Nursing and the Joint Commission on the Accreditation of Health Care Organizations. Her main consulting and research activities have focused on work redesign and care delivery models. She has published numerous articles and chapters on job design theory for professional service work, the Professionally Advanced Care Team (ProACT) model developed at RWJUH, integration of work redesign and shared governance, and evaluation research.

Tonges has served as a member of the board of directors of the Organization of Nurse Executives of New Jersey. She is a Commonwealth Fund Executive Nurse Fellow and a recipient of the American Organization of Nurse Executives' Nursing Administration Research award.

The Contributors

BRIAN J. ANDERSON is medical adviser for Cardiac Services at Unity and Mercy Hospitals in the Allina Health System in Minneapolis, Minnesota, and a director of the Allina Health System, chairing its Committee on Quality and serving on the governance, strategy, and finance committees. He serves on the finance committee of Mercy Health System in Farmington Hills, Michigan, and chairs the private sector relations committee of the Minnesota chapter of the American College of Cardiology. Anderson received his B.S. degree (1969) in physiology at the University of Minnesota and his M.D. degree (1973) from the University of Minnesota School of Medicine.

Anderson became a fellow of the American College of Cardiology in 1985. He founded Metropolitan Cardiology Consultants and currently is the managing partner. Anderson has been a consultant and lecturer for the Center for Case Management and coauthored and taught a curriculum on clinical pathways for the Joint Commission on the Accreditation of Healthcare Organizations.

ANN SCOTT BLOUIN is a partner with Ernst and Young's health care consulting practice and serves on the editorial board of the *Journal of Nursing Administration*. She has published extensively in the *Journal of Nursing Administration* and *Nursing Spectrum* and has coauthored chapters in several health care management textbooks. Currently, Blouin holds faculty appointments at the Joint Commission on Accreditation of Healthcare Organizations, Saint Xavier University, and DePaul University.

Blouin received her M.S.N. degree (1980) in nursing from Loyola University, her Ph.D. degree (1994) in nursing sciences and her M.B.A. degree (1994) concurrently from the University of Illinois at Chicago.

KATHLEEN A. BOWER is principal and co-owner of the Center for Case Management in South Natick, Massachusetts. She earned her B.S.N. degree (1968) from Georgetown University, her M.S.N. degree (1972) from Boston College, and her D.N.Sc. degree (1991) from Boston University.

Prior to her current role at the Center for Case Management, Bower held management and administrative positions over seventeen years at the New England Medical Center in Boston. In those roles, she was part of the team that invented the clinical path and provider-based case management technologies.

In her current role, Bower provides education and consultation about care management strategies throughout the United States and has done extensive international work. She has authored numerous publications on these topics as well and is on the editorial board of two journals.

BARBARA BUTURUSIS is a manager with Ernst and Young's health care consulting practice. She has over twenty-six years of health care experience and operational expertise in integrated delivery system service line administration, continuum of care operations, and care management.

Buturusis has published articles on geriatric care, home care, and self-directed work teams. Since joining Ernst and Young, she has worked on due diligence, contract management office, accreditation, and redesign engagements. She received her B.S.N. degree (1981) from Lewis University and her M.S.N. degree (1984) from Loyola University.

SHARON A. HENRY is director of Cardiovascular, Respiratory and Cardiovascular Nursing Services at Mercy and Unity Hospitals, of Allina Health System in Minneapolis, Minnesota. She also is a consultant for the Center for Case Management in South Natick, Massachusetts. She earned her B.S.N. degree (1981) at Anoka Ramsey Community College and her B.A. degree (1998) in Health Care Administration and Education at Metropolitan State University, Minneapolis, Minnesota.

Henry has presented at national and local conferences with a focus on health care management and product line leadership and has authored articles on case and care management, product line management and quality improvement. She has served as state director of the Minnesota Chapter of the Association of Clinical Cardiovascular Administrators and as president of the Anoka County Chapter of the American Heart Association, Minnesota Affiliate.

MARIA HILL is a senior consultant for the Center for Case Management. She earned both her B.S.N. (1979) and M.S.N. (1985) degrees at the University of Wisconsin–Madison. Her M.S.N. degree included a clinical focus in nephrology and a functional focus in administration.

Hill is a national speaker who creates and leads conferences on a variety of topics including CareMap, case management, disease management and panel management systems, the documentation-automation interface of the patient medical record across the health continuum, and the interface between variance management and continuous quality improvement.

Hill's articles and chapters on care management have appeared in a variety of journals and books, including *Managing Outcomes Through Collaborative Care: The Application of Care Mapping and Case Management.*

TERESA MIKENAS JACOBSEN is principal consultant and founder of Associates in Clinical Systems, a consulting practice that specializes in the integration of care delivery through technology and streategic change.

Jacobsen's work as a clinical informaticist began in the late 1970s with the implementation of one of the first hospital information and nursing management systems for a major academic medical center. She has published many papers and articles related to the clinical systems field.

Jacobsen is also an associate with the Center for Case Management and cofounder of the Midwest Alliance for Nursing Informatics (MANI). She received the Clinical Systems Award in 1995 from the Health Information and Management Systems Society (HIMSS), where she is a fellow, and has served on the HIMSS board of directors and the editorial boards for the *HIMSS Journal, Healthcare Information Management,* and *Computers in Healthcare* magazine.

JONATHAN KAPLAN is a partner and area director of East/Great Lakes Health Care Performance Improvement Consulting Services for Ernst and Young. Prior to joining Ernst and Young, Kaplan worked for a major health care information technology firm. He received his A.B. degree (1979) in economics from Cornell University and his M.P.H. degree (1980) from the University of Pittsburgh.

Kaplan is a frequent speaker at professional organizations as well as graduate education seminars. His presentations range from health care reform, repositioning health care for the future, and supporting the reengineering of health care through information technology.

BONITA ANN PILON is an independent health care consultant and associate professor at Vanderbilt University in Nashville, Tennessee. She earned her B.S.N. degree (1972) at Barry University, Miami, her M.S.N. degree (1975) at the University of Florida, Gainesville, and her Ph.D. degree (1988) in nursing administration at the University of Alabama, Birmingham. She has held several executive positions in health care organizations.

Pilon has consulted internationally on quality improvement, clinical pathways, and case management in the United Kingdom, Canada, and Singapore. She has also been the recipient of several demonstration grants in the areas of hospital-based and community-based case management and presents frequently at national conferences.

JOANNE RITTER-TEITEL is a health care consultant and a Ph.D. candidate at the University of Pennsylvania's Health Services and Policy Research Center in the School of Nursing. She received her B.S.N. degree (1977) from Columbia University and her M.A. degree (1985) in the delivery of nursing services from New York University. Prior to becoming a consultant, Ritter-Teitel was a full-time doctoral fellow at the University of Pennsylvania. Her research area of interest is clinical integration and its relationship to clinical outcomes.

As director of Critical Care Nursing at Robert Wood Johnson University Hospital from 1986 through 1993, Ritter-Teitel led the effort to develop the professionally advanced care team model for critical care (ProACT-CC), which received national and international attention. Her publications regarding this model have appeared in several journals.

Throughout her career, Ritter-Teitel has held adjunct faculty appointments at Rutgers University, Columbia University, and Johns Hopkins University. She serves on the editorial review board for the *Journal of Nursing Case Management*.

SUSAN ROBERTSON is a consultant in the health care practice of Coopers and Lybrant. She received her B.S.N. degree (1981) and M.S.N. degree (1989) in Medical Surgical Nurse Specialty from Adelphi University, Garden City, New York. Robertson's prior position was administrative director of Quality Management for North Shore Health System. She also has six years of case management experience and cofounded the Nassau-Suffolk Case Management Networking Alliance. She has coordinated multiple case management conferences, published several articles, and consults and lectures extensively on the topic.

ROBERT B. WILLIAMS is senior manager of Health Care Consulting at Ernst and Young. He received his B.A. degree (1972) from

Hampden-Sydney College, his M.D. degree (1976) from Medical College of Virginia, and his M.I.S. degree (1974) from Virginia Commonwealth University. Williams has served as associate clinical professor in the Department of Family Practice at the Medical College of Virginia and as adjunct faculty at the Department of Health Administration at Virginia Commonwealth University. He is a member of the American Academy of Family Physicians, the American College of Physician Executives, and the American Medical Association. His special interests include physician-driven health care enterprises, academic medical center organizations, and regulatory issues.

Clinical Integration

Part One

Framing Clinical Integration

Chapter One

Clinical Integration in Organized Delivery Systems

Responding to New Challenges in Health Care

Mary Crabtree Tonges

In health care today, clinical integration is a goal, not a reality. This book will help health care organizations develop practical applications of integrated delivery system theory, moving beyond the administrative merger phase and adding value as a system through clinical integration of their services.

As McEachern (1996, p. 1) has pointed out, there is a sense of urgency about moving forward with clinical integration because "You will not have the same amount of time as they had in California as managed care penetrated the market. You'll have months, not years, to react, and if you don't have an infrastructure ready, systems in place, you will lose."

What Is Clinical Integration, and Why Is It Important?

As Figure 1.1 shows, *clinical integration* is the degree to which preventive, diagnostic, and therapeutic care delivery processes are organized to achieve key clinical outcomes of individual patients and aggregate populations and to ensure smooth transitions within and across sites and over time.

McManis's (1990) foresightful prediction regarding the need for clinical integration in the nineties appears to be among the earliest uses of the term. Clinical integration is a key concept in cutting-edge health services administration theory and research (Conrad,

3

Figure 1.1. Clinical Integration.

The coordination of care delivery processes across
a continuum of time and location

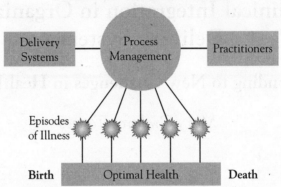

Developed by Brian Anderson, Allina Health Systems, Minneapolis, MN.

1993; Shortell, Gillies, Anderson, Mitchell, & Morgan, 1993;
Gillies, Shortell, Anderson, Mitchell, & Morgan, 1993; Shortell,
Gillies, Anderson, Erickson, & Mitchell, 1996).

A combination of factors—the collapse of national health care
reform, continuing market-driven reforms, and the growth in managed care—has led independent hospitals and other health care
facilities to form larger networks. To sustain a position in the managed care market, providers need capacity, location, and a full scope
of services. Moreover, the key to success in a capitated environment is disease management, which requires careful coordination
and continuity of care across the continuum. It is extremely difficult, if not impossible, to manage care effectively over time in a
fragmented delivery system. These requirements drive the restructuring of the health care industry.

The integration trend is reflected in the 1993 title change of
the journal of the American Hospital Association from *Hospitals* to
Hospitals and Health Networks. Yet creating network structures,
either through merger or contractual affiliation, is merely a first step
toward the ultimate goal of integration: a delivery system that can
provide quality care at a controlled cost. Integration is also an in-

ternal process. As Middlebrook (1996, p. 80) pointed out, "Merely assembling the pieces under one umbrella doesn't mean a system will operate as one. Within each operating unit are rules, traditions and cultures that can impede the smooth transition of patients from one setting to another."

While the integration of separate provider organizations into networks may be business-driven, the ability to coordinate care across a continuum of sites and services is what makes it patient-driven and profitable. Achieving coordination and continuity of care within an organized delivery system—clinical integration (Conrad, 1993; Gillies, Shortell, Anderson, Mitchell, & Morgan, 1993)—is the focus of this book. This chapter introduces the topic and provides an overview of the organization and content of the book.

Structural and Functional Integration: Necessary but Not Sufficient

Although both organizational and administrative integration are necessary steps in building an organized delivery system (Shortell, Gillies, Anderson, Mitchell, & Morgan, 1993), they are not sufficient to realize this strategy's potential for cost-effectiveness. In the rush to get into networks, organizations often engage in a frenzy of deal making. Arrangements are pursued with multiple partners simultaneously. Many contracts are signed out of fear that opportunities will pass by, and the hesitant will be left out of the flow of patients and revenues.

Some of these relationships become more important and lasting than others, and pundits liken these negotiations to courtship dance. "They are announcing that they are married, when really they are only engaged" (McEachern, 1995, p. 1). Extending this metaphor, clinical integration is like having a family: partners are inextricably linked in the creation of a new entity that requires long-term cooperative effort.

The fundamental goal of integration is to increase the value of the product. As Figure 1.2 illustrates, the value of health care can

Figure 1.2. Value in Health Care.

$$\text{Value} = \frac{\text{Quality} + \text{Service}}{\text{Price}}$$

be expressed as the ratio of quality of care and customer service to price. To better assess the value that providers deliver, employers and payers strive to develop more sensitive measures of quality, such as the Health Plan Employer Data and Information Set (HEDIS). This formula makes it clear that value can be increased by improving quality and service or by decreasing price.

Mergers and acquisitions may decrease the denominator by reducing administrative costs (by eliminating redundant positions, for example), but these are likely to be one-time savings. The real value lies in changing the variables—increasing the numerator and decreasing the denominator—through better coordination of care. Results from the Health Systems Integration Study (HSIS) (Shortell, Gillies, Anderson, Mitchell, & Morgan, 1993), a longitudinal investigation of regionally based networks, support the relationship between clinical integration and increased efficiency and profitability.

Although employers and payers are still very focused on price, as managed care markets continue to evolve and prices are driven to consistently low levels, quality will emerge again as a key competitive issue. Based on extensive research with patients, Gerteis, Edgman-Levitan, Daley, and Delbanco (1993) have identified seven dimensions that patients use in evaluating the quality of hospital care. Two of these dimensions—coordinating care and integrating services, and facilitating the transition out of the hospital—are encompassed within clinical integration. Thus clinical integration is synonymous with specific aspects of what these researchers describe as patient-centered care.

In summary, clinical integration is the win-win strategy that enables organized delivery systems to achieve their cost-quality objectives: improved coordination and continuity increase the quality of care, which in turn facilitates the management of cost.

Evolution of Clinical Integration

To date, health systems have evolved through four generations of development:

1. In the 1970s, loose affiliations of hospitals shared purchasing, insurance, and some financing.

2. In the 1980s, holding companies developed independent lines of business (such as managed care, ambulatory, and long-term care).

3. In the 1990s, business lines integrated locally, and physicians were brought into the mix to knit services into a continuum of care.

4. Today, systems are assuming financial risk and striving to demonstrate the added value of sharing best clinical practices across sites (Lumsdon, 1996b).

Clinical integration is an essential feature of organized delivery systems(Shortell, Gillies, Anderson, Mitchell, & Morgan, 1993), which have also been described as vertically integrated health systems (Conrad, 1993). *Vertical integration* can be defined as "the coordination of inputs (equipment, supplies, human resources, information, and technology) and intermediate outputs (preventive, diagnostic, acute, chronic, and rehabilitative services) to attain the end goal of optimal personal health" (Conrad, 1993, p. 491). Thus, vertically integrated health systems have the capacity to coordinate the care of individual patients over time. Although vertical integration suggests common ownership, coordination of care can also be accomplished within a system of contractual relationships, described by Goldsmith (1995, p. 11) as "virtual integration."

Integrated delivery system (IDS) theory, as developed by Shortell and colleagues (1993, 1996) and Conrad (1993), suggests that there are three dimensions of health system integration, and these dimensions develop at different times as a system matures. The dimensions can be described as follows:

1. *Administrative or functional integration* refers to the coordination of key administrative support functions and activities, such as planning, information systems, and financial management. This kind of integration occurs early in the process.

2. *Provider* or *physician-system integration* refers to physicians' identification with the system and involvement in shared accountability (including economic links, use of facilities and services, and involvement in planning, management, and governance). This integration also occurs early on. Physicians are currently the major group of providers, but other groups, such as nurse practitioners, may be included as reimbursement regulations change.

3. *Clinical integration*, again, refers to the coordination of patient care services across operating units within the system and builds on and develops after functional and provider-system integration.

Structural integration, which refers to the creation of the system relationships, may represent an additional dimension or phase at the beginning of the process.

Findings from the HSIS indicate that most systems are still in the early phases of the integration process (Lumsdon, 1995). Indeed, Shortell and colleagues (1996) have indicated that they prefer to describe these emerging delivery systems as organized rather than integrated, because very few, if any, current systems have achieved the end state of integration. Given the magnitude and complexity of the change integration represents, this is not surprising. In acute care during the seventies and eighties, poor communication and continuity between inpatient and ambulatory care within the same hospital was the norm. In the early nineties, few organizations owned or influenced a network of facilities providing a continuum of services, and even in those that did, there was generally little effort to coordinate care across sites or even a recognition of the need to do so.

In the mid to late nineties, many newly formed networks are striving to improve care coordination through initiatives such as clinical path[1] or CareMap and case management systems across several hospital sites. Implementing these programs in one hospital can be very challenging. Typical barriers range from clinicians and managers who dismiss the effort as an unimportant "nursing project" to those who actively resist what they perceive as a threat to their control. As demanding as this work can be in one facility, however, it is even more arduous to integrate the efforts of several hospitals, a Medical Services Organization (MSO), and managed care department. Moreover, the culture clashes, suspicion, and resentments frequently associated with merger and acquisition intensify the difficulties.

Zander has proposed that one reason why integration has progressed slowly in most systems may be the focus on starting with administrative and physician-system links, rather than starting with patients and working backward (personal communication, 1997). From this perspective, IDS theory may be more descriptive than prescriptive. In Zander's view, this approach results in integration issues being only partially addressed at each of the three levels: administrative, physician-system, and clinical.

This is an original and thought-provoking idea. Yet the dominant paradigm indicates that "it is not possible to create clinically integrated care without physicians who serve as the key decision makers in the process and without certain functions such as information systems and quality management in place" (Shortell, Gillies, Anderson, Erickson, & Mitchell, 1996, 40–41). Or as Anderson suggests in Chapter Three, the importance of the physicians' role cannot be overemphasized, and the extent to which practicing physicians play an integral role in governance and operations of a delivery system will largely determine its success. One solution to this dilemma may be to take a less linear approach and strive to develop elements of the three types of integration in concert.

Callaway (1997) has suggested that the development of the integrated delivery system concept and theory has "helped the industry organize its approach to integration around key concepts and tools" (p. 22). She also noted, however, that this is a practical area and stresses the need to consider both the appropriateness of integration strategies to local market conditions and the unique attributes of the organization in question. This book is designed to meet practitioners' needs by providing a useful blend of theory and practice, with an emphasis on real-world strategies and lessons from pioneers in the field.

Overview of the Book

Focusing on clinical integration within the context of organized delivery systems, the book's organizing framework is built around strategies for administrative and provider-system integration and practices to make clinical integration work.

Part One provides the reader with a good theoretical base for the strategies and practices that follow. Following this introductory chapter, Chapter Two offers a more comprehensive explanation of the theory of clinical integration and, very importantly, its managerial implications. Within the context of integrated delivery systems, clinical integration is described as the new fundamental necessity, with administrative and provider-system integration as necessary complements. Chapter Two reviews mechanisms for clinical integration and introduces business process reengineering as a mechanism for both administrative and clinical integration.

The chapters in Part Two summarize the infrastructure needed to support the practices explained in Part Three. Shortell and his colleagues (1996) have proposed that vision and culture are among the precursors of organized delivery systems. Writing about organizational culture as an integrator, Ummel (1997, p. 73) suggested, "The most powerful determinant of success over the longer term may be the most intangible ingredient." Chapter Three explains how the system's mission, vision, and shared values give rise to structure and behavior directed toward achieving systemwide goals. The author discusses the creation of a common clinical culture as a means of achieving clinical integration, with particular attention to the physician's perspective and role in this endeavor.

Building on the definitions in Part One, Chapter Four explains enterprisewide reengineering as a systems strategy to increase consistency and provide the infrastructure for both clinical and administrative integration. Application of these concepts and methods is depicted in a case study at the conclusion of the chapter. This example illustrates the use of spider diagrams, a new tool to assess managed care readiness ("Insider spider," 1997). These diagrams provide a tool for analyzing the fit between local market conditions, organizational attributes, and integration strategies. Such a fit is critical to success.

Chapter Five discusses product and service line structure as an administrative integration mechanism. The chapter details how an organizational structure based on product or service lines can facilitate coordination of patient care across delivery sites. Brian Anderson and Sharon Henry, authors of Chapters Three and Five respectively, lead the cardiac product line at Mercy and Unity Hospitals of the Allina Health System, and their partnership has been featured in a *Hospitals and Health Networks* cover story concerning the changing nature of nurse-physician relationships in a managed care environment (Lumsdon, 1996a). Based on its size, longevity, and degree of integration, Allina is among the eight systems recognized as leaders in the integration movement (Solovy, 1997).

Chapter Six addresses the challenges of physician-system integration. Paying particular attention to payment methods, the chapter describes a multifaceted approach to influencing physician behavior, which includes regulation, incentives, and feedback. The chapter also stresses the need for system administrators to understand clinicians' needs and to reach out to them in ways that respond to their immediate priorities.

Part Three includes four chapters that comprise the core of the book. Each of the chapters covers a specific approach or tool used to foster and strengthen clinical integration:

- Information systems
- Clinical path/CareMap tools
- Case management roles and systems[2]
- Common quality management and education

Chapter Seven describes the essential role information systems play in supporting care coordination and management across delivery sites. The chapter presents major issues in the development of integrated information systems and uses case studies to illustrate key points.

Chapter Eight outlines the lessons learned from a large organized delivery system that implemented CareMaps as a system-level clinical integration strategy. Specific objectives included a decrease in unnecessary variation in care for the same case types within a multihospital system (clinical standardization) and more coordinated, cost-effective care for patients across the system. The chapter describes the methods developed to achieve these objectives, including a systemwide variance analysis and management program, and plans for further vertical integration.

Chapter Nine presents an analysis of case management models for multiprovider systems, discusses the case manager role within an integrated delivery system, and outlines approaches to developing a case management program in this setting.

Chapter Ten describes how continuous quality improvement, outcomes management, and clinical education can be interrelated to form a powerful integrative engine. The chapter also discusses the role executive leadership and the governing board play in actualizing the combined potential of these clinical integration mechanisms.

Chapter Eleven presents my summary of the book's main themes and key points and suggests next steps. The following five themes are identified and discussed:

1. The changing nature and fundamental importance of relationships
2. The need for leadership
3. The rewards and risks of information technology
4. Multiple approaches and synergistic effects
5. The long view on payback from prevention

This concluding chapter emphasizes the need for ongoing systematic evaluation in three areas: (1) the outcomes of clinical integration, (2) the effects of suggested mechanisms on integration, and (3) the influence of specific approaches to implementing these mechanisms. I describe possible methods to assess the effects of clinical integration at the level of the case type and community. Again, organized delivery systems are an emerging phenomenon, and findings from such research will be critical to the future organization of health care delivery.

Content for Specific Audiences

Individuals with a broad interest in clinical integration are likely to need all chapters; however, other readers may be able to use the book more selectively. Within the practitioner group, there are several potential audiences for the book: (1) administrators who must set the stage for and encourage clinical integration, (2) physicians taking leadership roles in these initiatives, and (3) nurses assuming primary responsibility for designing and implementing clinical integration mechanisms.

Administrators may be most interested in the strategies outlined in Part Two; however, those who are unfamiliar with the tools may also find the detailed descriptions of practices in Part Three helpful. The importance of administrative leadership and what administrators' direction and support can lend or take away from clinical integration are presented in detail in Chapter Ten and referred to in Chapters Three through Nine.

Physicians may be most interested in Chapters Three and Six, which focus most directly on physician-system integration. Nurses who are primarily interested in implementation may find Chapter Five and Chapters Seven through Ten most valuable.

The Journey Toward Clinical Integration

This book takes a journey into the unfamiliar terrain of clinical integration in an effort to capture the essence of this concept where it lives: in the clinical environment. The goal is to make clinical integration real and to provide practical suggestions to make it work. Yet clinical integration is an elusive and challenging topic, and our study and understanding of it is in its infancy. Given these constraints, full answers do not yet exist, but the chapters that follow begin to address the following pressing questions:

- Does clinical integration really improve quality? Can we prove it?
- Does clinical integration cost less? More?
- What are the biggest challenges, threats, and opportunities?
- What is a good road map for a system to follow on its journey to clinical integration?
- How does a system know when it gets there?

Notes

1. There are several different types of clinical recommendations. In this book, the following definition of terms, compiled by Bergman (1994, p. 70), are used:

- *Clinical practice guidelines:* Adopted by the National Academy of Sciences' Institute of Medicine to refer to standards developed to assist practitioner and patient decisions about appropriate care in specific clinical circumstances (*Clinical Paths: Tools for Outcomes Management,* AHA, 1994).

- *Practice parameters:* Referred to by the AMA as educational tools that enable physicians to obtain the advice of recognized clinical experts, stay abreast of the latest research, and assess the significance of conflicting clinical research findings.

- *Critical pathways* or *clinical paths:* Clinical management tools that organize and time the major interventions of nursing staff, physicians, and other departments for a particular case type, subset, or condition.

- *CareMaps:* Second-generation clinical paths that show the relationships of sets of interventions to sets of intermediate outcomes along a time line, merging standards of care with standards of practice in a cause-and-effect relationship across time. (CareMap is a registered trademark of the Center for Case Management in South Natick, Massachusetts.)

2. Similar to the terminology for different types of clinical recommendations, there are several terms related to case management that should be differentiated. The following definitions developed by the Center for Case Management are used in this book:

- *Coordination of care:* Coordination of care is an umbrella term the encompasses several different, complementary strategies for managed care, including care and case management (see Figure 9.1).

- *Care management:* Refers to a unit-level accountability model in which every patient's care is managed by a specific nurse working with clinical path or CareMap tools.

- *Case management:* Refers to a clinical system that focuses on the accountability of an identified individual or group for coordinating a patient's care across the continuum of care. This approach is appropriate for management of the most complex patients (approximately 20 percent).

These terms are primarily used and further explained in Chapters Seven and Nine.

References

Bergman, R. (1994). Getting the goods on guidelines. *Hospitals and Health Networks, 68*(20), 70–74.

Callaway, M. M. (1997). Integration in the real world. *Healthcare Forum, 40*(2), 20–27.

Conrad, D. A. (1993). Coordinating patient care services in regional health systems: The challenge of clinical integration. *Hospital and Health Services Administration, 38*(4), 491–508.

Gerteis, M., Edgman-Levitan, S., Daley, J., & Delbanco, T. L. (Eds.). (1993). *Through the patient's eyes.* San Francisco: Jossey-Bass.

Gillies, R. R., Shortell, S. M., Anderson, D. A., Mitchell, J. B., & Morgan, K. L. (1993). Conceptualizing and measuring integration: Findings from the Health Systems Integration Study. *Hospital and Health Services Administration, 38*(4), 467–489.

Goldsmith, J. (1995). It's time for virtual integration. *Hospitals and Health Networks, 69*(7), 11.

Insider spider. (1997). *Hospital and Health Networks, 71*(7), 76–77.

Lumsdon, K. (1995). Watch for flying phrases. *Hospital and Health Networks, 69*(6), 79–82.

Lumsdon, K. (1996a). Dynamic duo. *Hospitals and Health Networks, 70*(21), 26–32.

Lumsdon, K. (1996b). Talk show. *Hospitals and Health Networks, 70*(14), 34–42.

McEachern, S. (1995). Heath systems begin clinical integration with oncology. *Health Care Strategic Management, 13*(4), 1, 19–23.

McEachern, S. (1996). Orthopedics one of easiest product lines to integrate. *Health Care Strategic Management, 14*(2), 1, 20–23.

McManis, G. L. (1990). Challenges of new decade demand break with tradition. *Modern Healthcare, 20*(2), 60.

Middlebrook, M. R. (1996). Some answers to the big questions in health care. *Modern Healthcare, 26*(42), 80.

Shortell, S. M., Gillies, R. R., Anderson, D. A., Mitchell, J. B., & Morgan, K. L. (1993). Creating organized delivery systems: The barriers and facilitators. *Hospital and Health Services Administration*, 38(4), 447–466.

Shortell, S. M., Gillies, R. R., Anderson, D. A., Erickson, K. M., & Mitchell, J. B. (1996). *Remaking health care in America*. San Francisco: Jossey-Bass.

Solovy, A. (1997). The health care 100. *Hospitals and Health Networks*, 71(6), 34–42.

Ummel, S. L. (1997). Pursuing the elusive IDN. *Healthcare Forum Journal*, 40(3), 73–76.

Chapter Two

Theory and Managerial Implications

Joanne Ritter-Teitel

The persistent economic burden of rising health care costs leads the newest power brokers—corporate and state purchasers of health care services—to pressure managed care organizations (MCOs) and health care providers to control costs. In turn, providers are searching for and experimenting with new, more cost-effective, coordinated systems of care that optimize clinical outcomes. In this era of care coordination and integration, the vision for optimizing clinical outcomes includes accountability for enhancing the population's overall health status. This vision may be a dream come true for health professionals who have sought to reduce fragmentation and better coordinate care.

This chapter describes the new fundamental necessity for clinical integration across health care organizations and care sites as the U.S. health care system strives to become cost-effective, coordinated, and outcome-driven. The chapter begins with a review of the evolution of integrated delivery systems (IDS). IDS are an important evolving organizational form that provide the structural framework for clinical integration.

Background

After President Bill Clinton's ambitious plan to reform the entire health care system failed to be legislated, Americans seemed to oppose comprehensive reform and instead favor incremental, local solutions to the nation's health care problems (Henry J. Kaiser Family Foundation, 1994). Indeed, without national legislation, local health care markets are accepting and enacting managed care strategies to transform the delivery of U.S. health care. Several states are pursuing aggressive health reform efforts targeted at controlling Medicaid costs by shifting the eligible population into managed care plans. At the national level, the federal government has taken similar measures to gently move the Medicare population into managed care.

Managed Care Penetration

Enrollment in MCOs continues to grow vigorously. Paul Ellwood, an originator of the health maintenance organization concept, asserts that managed care is no longer a model proposed for the U.S. health care system; rather, managed care *is* the health care system (Belkin, 1996). This may be an overstatement, but managed care is rapidly *becoming* the U.S. health care system.

Inpatient hospital days, a major target of MCOs, are shrinking. The reliance on expensive physician specialists has also been reduced. Primary care providers, as generalist gatekeepers, are charged with identifying health problems early, reducing the use and costs of expensive specialists, and avoiding costly hospital care.

MCOs have created a fierce economic pressure to bring all components of the health care delivery system together and create a point of accountability. Capitation, a prospective fixed reimbursement system, further intensifies the pressure to reduce costs by providing care in the most appropriate setting and keeping patients healthy.

Impact on Hospitals

The growing influence of managed care in local health care markets, with its cost and outcome imperatives, creates a need for fundamental reform of the U.S. health care system in general and acute care hospitals in particular. The following reductions in utilization have been forecasted for university hospitals: a 24 percent reduction in hospital patient days, 30 percent reduction in hospital revenues, and 30 percent decline in medical specialist revenues (Iglehart, 1995). The result of such changes is that the majority of hospitals either belong to or are developing integrated delivery systems as a means of protecting themselves against the increasingly challenging reimbursement environment.

The centrality of the hospital in the traditional U.S. health care system is well acknowledged; but the future position of the hospital is uncertain. In the evolving health care system, the force of managed care may push hospitals to the periphery. In another scenario, they may remain at the hub, but as entities of IDS in which acute care beds play only a modest role.

Integrated Delivery Systems

IDS offer a full range of services to patients and reduced transaction costs to purchasers. These systems are defined as "a network of organizations that provides or arranges to provide a coordinated continuum of services to a defined population and is willing to be held clinically and fiscally accountable for the outcomes and the health status of the population served" (Shortell, Gillies, Anderson, Mitchell, & Morgan, 1993, p. 447).

Much of our current understanding of IDS is derived from the Health Systems Integration Study (HSIS),(Gillies, Shortell, Anderson, Mitchell, & Morgan, 1993; Shortell, Gillies, Anderson, Mitchell, & Morgan, 1993). These researchers have made fundamental contributions to the theoretical and empirical understanding of IDS.

The IDS of today are distinctly different from the earlier systems developed in the late seventies and early eighties, which were actually horizontally linked hospital chains. Early hospital systems were designed to fulfill several objectives:

- Achieve economies of scale in joint purchasing
- Operate more efficiently by sharing information and clinical technology systems

- Share corporate management
- Enhance access to capital

Such loosely linked systems were designed to offer protection against changes in the reimbursement environment but not to improve the health status of the patient populations they served (Shortell, 1988). The reimbursement system paid for discrete episodes of care and lacked incentives to coordinate these episodes and improve the patient population's overall health status.

Sharing Risk

Unlike early hospital systems operating within a fee-for-service reimbursement environment, IDS operate in a managed care environment. The percentage of managed care penetration, while still varied across the country, is growing. In addition, IDS are increasingly operating in a performance-based reimbursement system that will require them to demonstrate their performance on the basis of improvement in the health and functional status of the population served relative to the costs incurred. If this broader responsibility for the population's health status becomes a widespread reality, IDS and their providers will assume unprecedented accountability for cost and patient outcomes. As the demand for improvement in clinical outcomes and health status grows, the IDS and their providers will be required to demonstrate empirically their differential impact on the health status of its community.

Danzon (1994), a health care economist, contends that while public policy should be watchful of these new networks abusing market power, they are our best hope of achieving a competitive and reasonably efficient solution to the challenge of providing high-quality health care at a reasonable cost. Growing anecdotal evidence suggests that care coordinated in and across sites achieves lower costs and better results for patients than fragmented, fee-for-service care (Lumsdon, 1995).

IDS Models

Many types of IDS organizational models are evolving, including those led by the hospital, the physician, and the MCO (Shortell, 1994). Within each type of model the organizational structures range from loosely to fully integrated.

Most IDS are led by the hospital and evolve due to the preexisting financial, organizational and leadership resources and expertise within hospitals. These pre-existing advantages are severely mitigated if the new IDS is unable to shift its emphasis from illness to the more contemporary health care management paradigm of wellness and disease prevention. No definitive data are available indicating which models are most effective in controlling costs and improving the quality of care across the network.

Attributes

IDS that are farther along the integration continuum tend to demonstrate common organizational attributes (Conrad, 1993; Shortell, Gillies, Anderson, Mitchell, and Morgan, 1993):

- A culture that emphasizes managing clinical and administrative activities across boundaries to create a seamless health care continuum
- An ability to conduct population-based needs assessments involving an epidemiological analysis of major employers, employees, and population groups served by the system
- Electronic linkages to clinical and financial data to connect patient and providers across the continuum of care
- Competency with continuous improvement processes to keep the large, potentially bureaucratic IDS responsive to its rapidly and ever-changing environment
- Networkwide incentive programs to reward systems thinking and activity

- Clinically integrated patient care management mechanisms that create systems thinking through clinical consensus and consistent care processes

Integration is characterized by the appropriate coordination of functions and activities across care sites and among other organizations in the same system. Thus, true system-level integration activities are interorganizational. While interorganizational integration is critical in an IDS, it is also difficult, which may explain why many systems do not consider themselves far along in system-level integration activities (Shortell, Gillies, & Devers, 1995). Shortell and colleagues report that those further along in interorganizational clinical integration activities demonstrate stronger financial results (Lumsdon, 1995).

While it seems logical that clinical outcomes would be optimized in highly integrated systems, commensurate with the enhanced access to services, reduced fragmentation and minimized duplication, these relationships have not yet been empirically demonstrated. However, integration intuitively seems the right course of treatment for our troubled health care system.

Dimensions and Mechanisms of Integration

There are three primary forms of integration: clinical, administrative, and provider-system (Gillies, Shortell, Anderson, Mitchell, & Morgan, 1993). These forms of integration are postulated to create the systems required to have an effect on the clinical outcomes and health status of the community that is served by the IDS. Integration, however, is the means for achieving high-quality health care—not the end. The ultimate outcome is improvement in the clinical and health status of the population served.

Clinical Integration

Clinical integration, the most important dimension of full integration, can be defined as the extent to which patient care services are coordinated across the various care sites, functions, and services

(Gillies, Shortell, Anderson, Mitchell, & Morgan, 1993). In our industry, the coordination of care for the individual patient over time is a fundamental goal; yet individual patient care coordination is no longer sufficient to meet the goals of evolving systems. Patterns and trends in individual care coordination must be aggregated to the system level to plan services for the entire member population. In other words, system-level data is essential to population-based care.

Clinical integration extends both horizontally and vertically. Horizontal integration constitutes the coordination of patient care services across care sites that are at the same stage of service delivery (Conrad, 1993; Gillies, Shortell, Anderson, Mitchell, & Morgan, 1993). Horizontal integration is often operationalized when two acute care hospitals merge or share clinical services. A new challenge, vertical integration, refers to the coordination of patient care activities across care sites that are at different stages of service delivery, such as coordinating care among primary care, hospital, and home care providers.

Strategies to strengthen clinical integration use mechanisms to link network care sites. These mechanisms include

- A single electronic medical record that is used by all network care sites
- Clinical decision support systems that produce credible, achievable, and user-friendly reports
- System-level clinical paths or practice guidelines that reflect clinical consensus
- Provider profiling and analysis of appropriate and inappropriate variations in practice patterns
- Transition planning strategies
- Case management programs for the patient population that tends to account for majority of the resource consumption
- Disease management programs for selected chronic conditions

- Demand management programs to help patients seek and select care at the most appropriate level and by the appropriate provider
- System-level continuous quality improvement initiatives
- System-level educational programming to foster learning and the development of a new system culture

These clinical integration mechanisms are designed to optimize patient outcomes by proactively planning care, reducing inappropriate variation among providers, linking disparate providers, and avoiding duplication or fragmentation across sites of care.

Clinical Integration Continuum

Clinical integration can be implemented at different levels. For example, hospital and enterprise and may be conceptualized as occurring along a continuum. Conrad (1993) identifies the following seven points along this continuum:

1. Coordinating episodic, hospital inpatient care
2. Linking general inpatient services to advanced or tertiary specialty care
3. Coordinating specialty services within the system
4. Linking acute and chronic services
5. Coordinating acute, chronic and rehabilitation services
6. Coordinating primary, secondary, and tertiary services
7. Coordinating care over an individual's entire health life cycle

This last point on the continuum may take decades to evolve as it requires portable health insurance policies that carry over from one job change to another. The rejection of Clinton's national health care plan in 1993 slowed the advancement of portable health insurance. Without fully portable insurance, the mammoth level of integration required to coordinate patient care for all members of the U.S. health care system, over their entire health life cycle, is more a dream than a realistic goal.

Administrative Integration

Administrative integration can be conceptualized as the extent to which key support functions and activities are coordinated across operating units. (Conrad, 1993; Gillies, Shortell, Anderson, Mitchell, & Morgan, 1993). This involves grouping people, work, and responsibilities so that boundaries do not divide patient care sites.

Early conceptualizations of integration argued that the clinical and administrative dimensions were parallel (Conrad & Dowling, 1990). More recent thinking suggests that clinical integration is a fundamental necessity, whereas administrative integration is its necessary complement (Conrad, 1993). Many hospitals are achieving some degree of intraorganizational administrative integration, for example, by organizing inpatient clinical services according to product lines. However, the new challenge is to create innovative new models at the system level.

There is a growing consensus that clinical integration is the hallmark characteristic of an IDS, and the focus of integrative efforts has shifted from administrative to clinical. Yet, the most successful IDS will manage both the clinical and administrative interconnections among care sites effectively. Administrative integration may lag behind clinical integration or vice versa; but as one form of integration gains momentum within the organization, mechanisms to strengthen the other will be needed. There are myriad administrative integration mechanisms that typically support clinical integration:

- Product line organizational structures
- Centralized human resource departments that provide consistent recruitment, performance measurement standards, and incentive programs

- Centralized information technology departments
- Centralized quality improvement departments

Provider-System Integration

The integration of a system and its providers (physicians and others) is the extent to which providers depend economically on the system, use the system's services and facilities, and actively participate in its planning, management, and governance (Gillies, Shortell, Anderson, Mitchell, & Morgan, 1993). Analysis of provider-system integration has focused on such issues as to the extent to which IDS medical staff share common goals and philosophies, participate in financial risk sharing, and use common guidelines for reviewing privileges and credentials across care sites.

The extent to which physicians are integrated into or collaborate with the system drives clinical integration. As Williams discusses in Chapter Six, the level of trust between physicians and hospitals is critical, and physician-system integration is further enhanced by appropriately aligned financial incentives, strong primary-specialist referral relationships, and clinical consensus.

One of the biggest challenges for IDS therefore is to develop the right mix of primary care providers and specialists spanning the service continuum. In the increasingly common gatekeeper role that they play, primary care physicians are critical customers of hospitals because they control referrals to specialists and the places where patients receive care.

A New Perspective

The transformation of a stand-alone hospital to membership in an IDS requires a strikingly different perspective. The components of this new perspective are summarized in Table 2.1 (Shortell, Gillies & Devers, 1995). Again, hospital-based health care professionals

Table 2.1. Shifts in Perspective from Hospital to IDS.

Hospital	⇒	Integrated Delivery System
Discrete episodes of inpatient care	⇒	Continuum of care
Treating illness	⇒	Promoting health
Caring for individual patients	⇒	Health status of defined populations
Commodity product	⇒	Value-added services
Market share of admissions	⇒	Covered lives
Fill the beds	⇒	Provide care at the appropriate level
Manage an organization	⇒	Manage an enterprise
Manage a department	⇒	Manage a market
Coordinate services	⇒	Actively manage and improve quality

Source: Adapted from Shortell, Gillies, & Devers, 1995.

must understand that the new emphasis on primary care is intended to improve the health status of the population served, not to fill hospital beds.

Executive leadership teams, as Pilon suggests in Chapter Ten, are encouraged to provide a clear vision for the mission of the IDS and the design of clinically integrated care models. This committed executive vision has many requirements for its models:

- They must use multidisciplinary collaborative approaches for development and maintenance.
- They must provide individual and systemic patient care coordination.
- They must be population-based and consider improving the health status of the community served.
- They must provide a seamless continuum in which care is provided in the most appropriate setting.

Although IDS are more easily visualized than operationalized, a clear vision and mission are key to the business process reengineering required to build an IDS.

Business Process Reengineering

Reengineering employs information technology to change core business processes radically with the goal of improving customer satisfaction and increasing efficiency and effectiveness. IDS are made up of five core business processes:

1. Assessing and securing the patient population
2. Care and service delivery
3. Outcome demonstration
4. Education and research
5. Enterprise management

Reengineering also involves transforming subprocesses that enable or limit clinical, administrative, and provider-system integration (such as the transformation of admission, discharge, and transfer into transition management).

At the heart of business process reengineering in an IDS is clinical reengineering, which is conceptualized as the design and implementation of innovative strategies to change care and service delivery and enhance the value to customers; that is, to improve the cost-effectiveness and outcomes of care delivery (Nackel, 1995). In an IDS, processes cross the service continuum, including acute, chronic, and wellness services. This work is difficult because it challenges traditional philosophies of care delivery and the values of health care professionals. Specifically, this process requires systems thinking among professionals affiliated with separate entities who must work together toward a common goal. This approach is unusual in a cottage industry that has traditionally praised professionals in the organization for their individual performance.

In clinical reengineering the design of process, people, and technology is integrated and holistic in order to actualize clinical integration across the care continuum. Processes also must be reengineered to support administrative and provider-system integration, which will in turn enhance clinical integration.

Forces Influencing Clinical Integration

There are political, organizational, and market forces affecting clinical integration in an IDS. Political forces including issues of ownership, policy, and sponsorship should be considered by those who assume responsibility for creating clinical management systems.

Political Factors

IDS ownership may influence the vision and enactment of clinical integration in the system. Conrad (1993) argues that clinical integration is possible without ownership of all organizations and care sites in the IDS, but common ownership facilitates clinical integration and care coordination.

An IDS may align or partner with other organizations rather than own them. It is more challenging to achieve clinical integration in an aligned IDS because this type of network is not likely to use traditional and uniform control measures, such as authority and system-level compensation and incentive programs, to influence the professional staff. Regardless of ownership, clinical integration strategies are the same in each corporate structure.

Another political issue that influences clinical integration is the extent to which the organizational structure allows each operating unit to remain decentralized, maintain its own governance, and continue its current management and clinical practices. While clinical integration strategies tend to be similar regardless of ownership, it is the administrative and provider-system integration strategies that may be quite different given the response to political issues.

Organizational Factors

While political issues are important, successful clinical integration can be facilitated by other organizational and market factors:

- Development of a network of primary care providers
- Extension of the breadth of services the institution offers
- Intraorganizational care management strategies

This last factor is particularly important. Most early clinical integration strategies (such as clinical paths and case management) were hospital-focused and initiated by nurses (Ethridge, 1987; Zander, Etheredge, & Bower, 1987). Although these care coordination strategies have received considerable attention in the literature, most of the reports have been anecdotal.

Despite the lack of rigorous research to date examining the link between clinical integration programs and patient outcomes, it appears that those organizations that have implemented internal clinical integration mechanisms and have a strong, committed vision for the system will be more facile in the creation of innovative system-level programs.

Market Factors

Two major market factors that influence the integration of clinical services are the penetration of managed care contracting and the advancement of information technology. The penetration of managed care in the local health care marketplace and its level of capitation is a market factor that has created a chain of organizational actions outlined earlier in this chapter. The more advanced the penetration of managed care in a local health care market, the more likely an IDS will engage in clinical integration activities. In addition, the advancement of clinical information systems to support the provision of care and single electronic medical records significantly enable clinical integration in an IDS. Sophisticated information systems play a central role in IDS ability to measure clinical integration and assess its effects.

Measuring Clinical Integration

Devers and her colleagues (1994) argue that the development of systemwide metrics of clinical, administrative, and provider-system integration may help overcome barriers to network formation and actually aid the development of systems thinking. The very process of developing, collecting, and analyzing systemwide indicators of clinical integration helps the IDS foster an operating unit's reconceptualization of its activities in system's terms. Assessments of individual operating units are viewed in terms of their individual performance *and* how they contribute to the system as a whole.

Certain proxy measures are currently used to assess clinical integration across care sites (Devers et al., 1994):

1. Clinical practice guidelines or path development
2. Uniformity of patient medical record
3. Clinical outcomes data collection and utilization
4. Clinical programming and planning efforts
5. Shared clinical support services
6. Shared clinical service lines

As previously suggested, clinical integration mechanisms that are intraorganizational are useful precursors of interorganizational clinical integration and should also be considered and measured.

These areas are considered starting points. As the measurement work continues, it should become possible to identify those mechanisms with the greatest leverage for achieving clinical integration. More importantly, there is a need to move beyond assessing the extent to which these mechanisms are in place and focus instead on the outcomes they are intended to achieve. As outcomes research methodologies increase in sophistication, such outcomes standards will include indicators of community health status, such as work and school attendance, as well as member satisfaction with the coordination of care.

Conclusion

Clinical integration within an IDS is an organizational form that is expected to meet the challenges of the evolving health care system in a way that traditional stand-alone health care organizations have been unable to do. A number of intraorganizational clinical integration mechanisms have been developed; building on this work, the creation of interorganizational mechanisms is in the beginning stages. As providers experiment with new, more cost-effective, coordinated systems of health care, we will have an unprecedented opportunity to add value through the improvement of the health and functional status of all Americans.

References

Belkin, L. (1996, December 8). But what about quality? *The New York Times Magazine*, p. 68.

Conrad, D. A. (1993). Coordinating patient care services in regional health systems: The challenge of clinical integration. *Hospital and Health Services Administration, 38*(4), 491–508.

Conrad, D. A., & Dowling, W. L. (1990). Vertical integration in health services: Theory and managerial implications. *Health Care Management Review, 15*(4), 9–22.

Danzon, P. M. (1994). Merger mania: An analysis. *Health Systems Review, 26*(6), 18–28.

Devers, K. J., et al. (1994). Implementing organized delivery systems: An integration scorecard. *Health Care Management Review, 19*(3), 7–20.

Ethridge, P. (1987). Nurse accountability program improves satisfaction, turnover. *Health Progress, 5,* 44–49.

Gillies, R. R., Shortell, S. M., Anderson, D. A., Mitchell, J. B., Morgan, K. L. (1993). Conceptualizing and measuring integration: Findings from the Health Systems Integration Study. *Hospital and Health Services Administration, 38*(4), 467–489.

Henry J. Kaiser Family Foundation/Harvard School of Public Health (1994). *News release: Post-election survey.* Menlo Park CA: Author.

Iglehart, J. K. (1995). Rapid changes for academic health centers: Second of two parts. *New England Journal of Medicine, 332*(2), 407–411.

Lumsdon, K. (1995). Watching for flying phrases. *Hospitals and Health Networks, 69*(6), 79–82.

Nackel, J. G. (1995). Breakthrough delivery systems: Applying business process innovation. *Journal of Society of Health Systems, 5*(1), 11–22.

Shortell, S. M. (1988). The evolution of hospital systems: Unfulfilled promises and self-fulfilling prophesies. *Medical Care Review, 45*(2), 177–214.

Shortell, S. M. (1994, March). The challenges of health care reform: Creating organized delivery systems. Paper presented at Integrated Service Networks Under Health Care Reform: Theory and Practice.

Shortell, S. M., Gillies, R. R., Anderson, D. A., Mitchell, J. B., & Morgan, K. L. (1993). Creating organized delivery systems: The barriers and facilitators. *Hospitals and Health Services Administration, 38*(4), 447–466.

Shortell, S. M., Gillies, R. R., & Devers, K. J. (1995). Reinventing the American hospital. *Milbank Quarterly, 73*(2), 131–160.

Zander, K., Etheredge, M. C., and Bower, K. A. (1987). *Nursing case management: Blueprints for transformation.* Boston: New England Medical Center.

Part Two

Strategies for Clinical Integration

Chapter Three

Values and Value

Perspectives on Clinical Integration

Brian J. Anderson

Up to this point, the book has broadly outlined the big picture of clinical integration within the context of integrated delivery systems (IDS). This chapter begins a more specific discussion of clinical integration strategies.

Amazing changes have occurred in health care delivery over the span of my career as a practicing physician. Upon leaving Internal Medicine residency in the mid-seventies, I and my colleagues entered a world where fee-for-service medicine flourished, outcomes research was primitive, information systems did not inform, length of stay was unheard of, and a clinical path had never been seen. Hospital systems did not exist as systems, HMOs were not yet heavyweights, more was better, and collaboration was a political transgression. Medical staffs were organized strictly by department; hospital managers functioned in silos; communication was by memo; and we were all woefully ignorant of the multidimensional aspects of quality in health care.

What a difference a decade or two makes! Our socioeconomic environment has forced the health care industry and health care providers to address change as never before. A large part of the change involves trying to deliver care in ways and places that we never have before and maximizing the efficiency and effectiveness with which we do it.

In this chapter I present integration through the eyes of a practicing clinician. In the role of internist and later cardiologist, I have participated in change at the level of direct patient care. From my role as a clinical program adviser in a community hospital has come the experience of the joys and frustrations of developing and implementing interdisciplinary collaborative practice initiatives. In my role as a board member of a succession of health care delivery systems that has culminated through mergers in the Allina Health System in Minnesota, I have helped address issues of mission, public policy, system development and integration, resource allocation, strategy, quality, physician relationships, and culture. Finally, as a consultant in case and care management, I have been able to see and hear directly from all types of health care professionals in all types of settings about their efforts to initiate and manage change.

This experience has convinced me that clinical integration is the logical centerpiece in the evolution we are all undergoing. Clinical integration focuses the attention, effort, and resources of health care organizations exactly where they must be focused for us to fulfill our collective professional obligation to the individuals and communities we serve.

The Environment

Health care in the Twin Cities of Minneapolis and St. Paul has been radically reshaped in response to social and economic forces. While in some respects the reshaping is qualitatively similar to that in many parts of the country, in other respects it is unique. Intense downward pressure on hospital bed occupancy has resulted in the closure of over one-third of the urban hospitals. The financial realities of declining reimbursement, high demand for capital, and duplication of services has helped to spur institutional collaborations and mergers.

The net result has been the emergence of a few dominant systems in a highly competitive marketplace. One of the major systems has joined with the university hospital in a complex arrangement that is being watched with great interest. One of the largest systems, Allina, has an insurance component with approximately one million covered lives. The entire HMO industry remains by law not-for-profit—Minnesota is the only state in the union where this is the case.

Managed care penetration is extremely high, yet discounted fee for service, rather than capitation, is the usual physician payment method. The major delivery systems, with their focus on primary care, have used physician practice acquisition as a strategy, but the actual number of owned physicians is relatively small. Staff model HMOs employ many physicians and are influential in the marketplace, but many have contracted clinics and physicians as affiliates in order to expand their geographic influence and improve access.

In response to the perceived consolidation of power in the dominant systems, several major corporations have developed an initiative to contract directly with caregivers, bypassing the insurance function and attempting to share risk and reward directly. A multiplicity of physician and physician-hospital organizations has formed, with varying success, to maintain or expand influence. Regional and rural hospitals struggle with the same issues as their urban colleagues, often with additional concerns unique to their size and location. Overlaying this complex organizational landscape is a powerful social consciousness and political will to ensure access to high-quality health care at an affordable cost to all residents of the state.

I have quickly sketched this environment to give you a sense of the complex world within which delivery systems and caregivers must navigate as they struggle with the issues of integration that are crucial to their success. In reality, nearly all of the delivery systems rely on providing service to patients enrolled in competing health plans, and most physicians work with or for several competing organizations and have contracts with multiple payers. While the various organizations describe themselves as systems, how much true integration and systematic behavior exists and is demonstrated is quite variable. A confounding factor that arises from this complex environment is that in order for any organization to be truly integrated and systematic in its behavior, it must often collaborate with its competitors. This is illustrated by the need for an HMO owned by one system to have contracts with providers and hospitals of competing systems in order to offer the range of choice that is a crucial marketing strategy. Although my environment has its unique features, health care organizations and providers across the country face many similar issues.

Why Integrate?

When considering integration, it has been helpful to think about the end results of work in terms of service, financial, and clinical outcomes. If I or my organization is to be successful, we must understand how closely interrelated these areas are. We must devise ways within the limits of our resources to minimize duplication and waste, to measure accurately the results of our work, and to use those measures to improve performance in all areas. Everyone involved in the work must understand very clearly what we are trying to accomplish, and everyone must have a sense of value in the process. This issue speaks directly to collaboration and integration and demands that we know where we're going before we start out—or that we at least think about it. In my experience as a care management consultant, I have been surprised by how many initiatives are launched without clearly defined goals and, consequently, no meaningful measures of success. As the King of Siam said, " 'Tis a great puzzlement!"

Mission Moves You

In order for any organization to achieve the type of integration necessary for success, there must be a fundamental understanding of what the organization is trying to accomplish and how it wants to accomplish it. Everyone in the organization must share this understanding, as it is the basic ingredient in building a viable culture that nurtures and promotes the work that achieves organizational goals.

This understanding begins not with a mission statement but with a carefully constructed statement of values. That statement of values cannot be handed down from on high but must be the distillation of input from all segments of the organization. Developing a process that allows physicians, managers, line workers, board members, and executives from across the organization to help craft the statement of values is a first step in building a culture of participation upon which functional and clinical integration must rest. The statement of values also provides a framework for decision making that is consistent, ethical, widely understood within the organization, and used not only in business units but at the bedside and in the boardroom. Because it is consistent and widespread, the value statement becomes a powerful integrating tool.

Many mission statements don't work, because either they don't reflect the values of the organization, they were written in a vacuum, or they are not based in the reality of an organization's environment and abilities. A well-developed mission statement can become the focal point around which integrative efforts revolve; in fact, it should be *the* focal point. A careful analysis of the health care needs of the individuals and communities served will identify not what our perception of those needs is but what theirs is. Ask them! An attentive ear to the needs of public health agencies, public policy bodies, regulators, special needs populations, and caregivers will help to round out a deep understanding of what the organization's "customers" desire. Then, in the context of the organization's resources, a meaningful statement of mission can be made. Knowledge and understanding of that statement must then be driven down and across the organization, so that everyone can understand where they are going and why. The mission and values absolutely must become part of everyone's consciousness, so that there is an everyday awareness of purpose. Executives and managers have the highest obligation to lead by voice and lead by example—visibly and forcefully exhibiting in their behavior how the organization's values and mission shape the way the work gets done.

The result of using values and mission as the basis for everyday work and decision making is progress toward building the common clinical culture that is so vital to integration. Part of the common culture, derivative from values and mission, is a shared desire to meet the clearly stated goals and objectives of the organization. But take note—the shared desire is a result of a participative and collaborative process of setting the goals. This requires on the part of the delivery system a deep understanding of the perspectives of all who will share in the work. Particularly with reference to physicians, it requires knowledge of the professional and economic concerns that a complex and rapidly changing environment has created. On the part of physicians, it requires a broadened appreciation of the social and economic factors operative in health care today. Only through this mutual knowledge and understanding can consensus be built around goals and strategies.

If a common culture is to be nourished and strengthened, two essential ingredients must be present: trust and accountability. Without these, an organization will be forever dealing with damage control in its relationships with providers and employees, waiting for work to be done, incurring the costs of poor quality, and generally wasting time and resources. I have often seen the negative effects on performance that occurred because no one was clearly accountable for a project; I have seen initiatives die because people did not trust each other enough to share information or resources. Without the ability to create and maintain trust and accountability, efforts at integration will be severely hampered, if not made impossible. But if a health care delivery system develops a culture of value-based decision making and has a clearly stated mission with goals and objectives that derive from it, then trust and accountability can also become part of "how we do our work."

The Physician Question

If we accept, as I believe we should, that clinical integration is the centerpiece of a successfully integrated delivery system, then surely physicians are key players. The question that bedevils many system administrators is, How do we get physicians to understand and participate in integration? As I noted in the preceding section, the prerequisite is the effort to build a common clinical culture. From that base, all other efforts relating to physicians can proceed.

Most systems must deal with physicians who are in private clinical practice, are often competing with each other, and work in a variety of practice structures. They must also deal with the tension between independent practices and those that may be owned or managed by a system. Even within staff model organizations, it is often difficult to get physicians to buy into and participate in clinical integration activities.

In my experience, the basic issues for physicians revolve around four key areas: access to patients, professional autonomy, reimbursement, and a lack of understanding that creates mistrust. I want to describe the reorganization and reengineering that logically occurs as a common culture is built around values and mission, for many of the solutions to the physician question (and other questions) lie in those processes.

The Building Blocks of Integration

There are six areas of critical importance to an integrated system based on a common culture:

1. Innovative and effective governance
2. Collaborative management
3. Collaborative practice
4. Team concepts and shared learning
5. Continuous performance improvement
6. Physician leadership and integration

Let's take a look at each of these in turn.

Governance

Systems that are truly integrated deliver health care services across a wide range of locations and time. They necessarily interact with myriad private and public agencies and with multiple care providers and payers. At each level of interaction, from corporate board to local organization, the composition and philosophy of the governance structures is of utmost importance.

At the corporate board level, for example, inclusion of health care consumers can bring to the table a skill set and depth of knowledge that will be extremely useful in examining community and consumer needs. People active in community agencies or volunteerism can offer a unique perspective. Increasingly, corporate boardrooms are being filled with physicians; in some instances they hold a near majority of seats and often occupy the chair and key committee posts. This diverse composition allows a board to gain deeper and wider knowledge as it moves down the path of integration. But regarding this arrangement I offer a word of caution: in order for such a diverse board to be successful, every effort must be made to avoid constituency-based appointments. Board members should be able to think broadly, avoid personal representational agendas, and be fully supportive of the organization's values and mission. They must be effective ambassadors for the change agenda. All too often the temptation to appoint a board member based on their constituency rather than their skills has resulted in poor performance.

Of particular importance are the governance structures hidden further down in the organization, closer to the point of care. These might deal with such activities as collection and use of clinical performance data, or development and management of a systemwide steering committee around a specific clinical discipline. In each instance, careful composition of the governance structure and function offers a chance to build trust and demand accountability—our two key ingredients for successful integration.

To illustrate, a major care delivery system I work with provides cardiovascular services at multiple hospitals within the system and has several competing physician groups. Each institution has its own cardiac services program managers and develops its own strategy and business plan based on its needs. There is limited ability to share financial and clinical outcomes data between sites. Because each site develops and implements its own programs, there is substantial duplication of effort and lack of awareness. Efforts to develop common clinical practice guidelines and clinical pathways have been difficult to coordinate. In an effort to address these issues (which are issues of integration), managers and practitioners from the multiple sites formed a systemwide steering committee. The committee was composed of managers and physicians who do work in cardiovascular care, including information systems and finance representatives. The committee's role was to provide a governance function for efforts to integrate cardiovascular services throughout the system. They sponsored a systemwide series of collaborative workgroups to develop and promulgate best practice recommendations around several cardiovascular disease states, including advice to senior management regarding public education, primary and secondary prevention, and common outcome measures. Through this process, trust is being built, learning shared, and resources focused in a more efficient way.

Regardless of the level at which the innovative and effective governance occurs, it should serve to build and maintain the common clinical culture of the system.

Collaborative Management

Executives and managers within an integrated delivery system will be faced with the challenge of structural reorganization that will promote integrated strategic planning, sharing of information, development of common performance measures, and disciplined resource allocation. A rigidly hierarchical organization will find it difficult to achieve maximum effectiveness and efficiency of operations, as it lacks the flexibility required to respond quickly to a fluid environment. An innovative and flexible structure will allow managers and executives to get closer to the point of care, which I believe is a key component in the development of a common clinical culture. When line workers, physicians, nurses, and operating unit personnel are at the same table with senior managers on a regular basis and are sharing in the work of the organization, two very powerful integrating forces can be unleashed. The first is the sense of worth and empowerment that caregivers and others will feel if their ideas, attitudes, and accomplishments are visibly valued by their "bosses." Loyalty to the mission and values of the organization is enhanced, and great energy is tapped to attain goals and objectives. The second result is that executives and senior managers begin to develop a deeper knowledge of their organization, its capabilities and limitations—they hear it directly from the people who do the work. This visible participation and listening, if it is followed by consistent value-based decision making, once again helps to build and strengthen the common culture.

A community hospital I visited as a consultant provides a case in point. Some members of the staff were trying valiantly to promote a modest level of clinical integration in the inpatient setting in order to remain competitive in their marketplace. Their length of stay and cost per case were not optimal, and they were trying to introduce case management and clinical paths as tools. A traditional medical and nursing staff structure was in place that appeared to be relatively rigid. A single person was designated as the case management and quality improvement "department" and charged with implementation. During my visit, various vice presidents made brief appearances at what were to be interdisciplinary meetings. As I visited with the CEO, he exhibited almost no knowledge of the initiative. There was no budget for the case manager to operate with; there was no clearly stated set of goals; and the board of directors was totally removed from the whole process.

Compare that scenario with another system where I observed that, based on the success of one or two operating units in reducing length of stay, cost per case, and inappropriate variation in frequency of procedures through the use of interdisciplinary teams and case management tools, corporate senior management made it a systemwide priority to share the learning and develop similar efforts at all operating units. Vice presidents routinely participated in the work, and the successes of the organization were known all the way to the corporate board.

For functional and clinical integration to move forward, collaborative management must also occur outside the walls of hospitals. To begin truly to identify and address the health issues of individuals and populations and to make the most effective and efficient use of resources, management in private clinics, public health agencies, schools, volunteer organizations, and long-term care facilities must be brought together. Recognizing that each has its own perspective, goals and resources, innovative delivery systems can be a catalyst to develop a common agenda that promotes clinical integration. The talents and resources of all concerned can be leveraged to have a synergistic effect on the health status of those served. Each organization will be able to advance its own cause, but ideally within a new context. This collaborative management will demand that the values and mission of each participant be honored and that there be discipline in the allocation of resources, with rigor in the appropriate use of outcome measures.

In the integrated delivery system of the future, the mark of effective management will not only be the ability to manage a hospital and its support structures but the ability to forge innovative and valuable relationships with other parties.

Collaborative Practice

Inherent in the concept of clinical integration, collaborative practice should be understood to encompass every level of activity within a delivery system. While there are clearly defined models of the most visible types of collaborative practice—such as multidisciplinary care teams—it is too often identified only with hospital-based patient care. In fact, the full expression of collaborative practice not only exists at that level but permeates the entire system.

Whether considering activity based on disease management, case management, preventive services, strategic planning, public health initiatives, or business plan development, the concept remains the same: by bringing together all of the people who have a legitimate interest in the enterprise in an environment that promotes constructive interchange, a wealth of energy and creativity can be focused on the work at hand in a way that is not otherwise possible. By properly managing that environment and the processes involved in accomplishing the work, and by continually testing decisions against the values and mission of the organization, a culture of trust and accountability can be strengthened.

Collaborative practice demands flexibility and a willingness to share knowledge. It is not about power or control, although these may lurk beneath a facade of cooperation. A favorite expression I have heard is "check your title at the door." Unfortunately, collaboration can also take on the pejorative hue of consorting with the enemy, especially among physicians. Cooperation is not capitulation!

Eliminating structural barriers to collaboration is extremely important. Barriers exist within and between the departments of hospital management, the operating and business units in a system, and between the system and those outside it. Barriers to collaboration also exist between physicians, practices, and hospitals. A key component in addressing these barriers is, once again, a clear understanding of the values, mission, and goals of the delivery system.

I have observed that the three most common barriers to collaborative practice are power, time, and money. Power flows not just from control but from a perception of authority and the ability to influence decision making. The amount of time anyone will devote to collaborative efforts is directly proportional to their perception of its value to them. Resource allocation and compensation are usually integral to some part of perceived value for time and work expended. These three barriers must be recognized and dealt with explicitly.

The most powerful tools for promoting collaborative practice are clearly stated values, mission, and goals, supported by effective management and caregiver leadership. Physicians play a key role as caregiver leaders, but so should nurses and other direct caregivers. Carefully selected and developed leaders who will "walk the talk" and set the standards of collaborative practice as everyday routine are the most valuable resource an integrated system can have.

I was recently involved in an excellent example of the power of collaborative practice. Two community hospitals within the same delivery system identified congestive heart failure as a high-volume, high-cost diagnosis. There was an unacceptably high readmission rate, while length of stay and cost per case issues were problematic. Additionally, there was wide variation in coding practices and treatment. All of these issues were identified by a cardiovascular services program team consisting of a program director, medical advisor, payor representative from the system health plan, members from data quality (which included medical record and information systems support), and finance. The findings of this team were presented to a full interdisciplinary cardiac services work team, which functioned in lieu of a department and included representatives from cardiology, internal medicine, surgery, anesthesia, pharmacy, nursing, rehabilitation, home care, chaplaincy, finance, and data quality. An action plan was devised that created a subgroup charged with developing an integrated inpatient-ambulatory clinical path, a clinical practice guideline with a preprinted order set, pilot projects with several clinics to implement the path, and a set of outcome measures. Leadership for the subgroup was provided by the medical advisor, and support services were supplied by the cardiovascular program office. Relationships were established with several clinic managers and their lead physicians, and clinic nursing staff were included on the work team. One of the clinics had a large capitated population, and data regarding the impact of this diagnosis on their financial performance provided a compelling argument for them to participate in the process. The health plan, recognizing congestive heart failure as a significant resource drain, was willing to alter payment methodologies to promote new practices aimed at reducing readmission.

The net result to date of this work in progress has been the establishment of a joint management committee with the large multidisciplinary clinic around all of cardiac services; creation of a coordinated inpatient-outpatient clinical path that includes handoffs to home care as well as expedited hospital-to-clinic discharge information; an outcome set including clinic and physician-specific measures; and creation of in-clinic consultation and exercise therapy provided by the hospital-based cardiovascular program. In the multispecialty clinic pilot, readmissions have decreased by over 75 percent, resulting in a net saving of over $500,000 to the clinic and the health plan. The cost accounting system used in hospital allows DRG-specific tracking of inpatient use of drugs, laboratory and radiology services, and other diagnostics by ordering physician as the sorting marker. Resource consumption can be cross-referenced to recommendations in the practice guideline for use as an educational tool to manage practice variation. Ambulatory care costs are monitored by the clinic and its health plan. Everyone, including the patient, has won through collaborative practice.

Team Concepts and Shared Learning

Have you ever heard of a basketball group? There's a good reason that you haven't—teams work together, groups get together. Absolutely crucial to the success of clinical and other types of integration is the concept of teams that work together and share what they learn. The value of the team lies in its ability to develop roles and accountabilities and to share work and its outcomes—be they successes or failures. Just as a basketball team has shooters, rebounders, and shot blockers, along with contributors who come off the bench, so a health system care delivery team, as it defines its goals and the work necessary to achieve those goals, can develop clear expectations of all its members based upon skills and competencies. The team members will be drawn from all areas within the scope of the collaborative practice necessary and can recruit members on an as-needed basis.

The team concept has major implications for the structure of health care systems and for the philosophy of how information and learning is shared. Some systems, in order to maximize flexibility and integrative capability, are drastically reshaping their management structures. Some hospital medical staffs are eliminating rigid departmental designs and organizing multidisciplinary teams around disease management concepts. Innovative nursing departments are developing ongoing clinical action teams that focus on a case or disease type in support of a larger product line or program-focused approach. Managers and caregivers from private clinics and other care delivery points are being recruited to be active participants. The common theme of the team approach is to draw on the talent assembled and push the learning down and across the entire organization. Strategies for the dissemination of information within the organization must be developed in order to perpetuate the spirit of teams and collaborative practice, and those strategies must be appropriately governed. Although some types of information of high strategic value must be closely held, many of the learnings in health care are appropriately viewed as nonproprietary and should be widely shared. A distinguishing characteristic of a highly integrated delivery system will be its ability to maximize learning experiences and effectively share them internally and externally. A particularly distinguishing trait will be the ability to use that learning to improve continuously.

Continuous Performance Improvement

Why don't I say continuous quality improvement? Continuous performance improvement is a dimension of quality and a very important cultural feature that integrated systems must approach with strategies appropriate for the location and audience. The concept of continually striving to perform at a higher level is an easier sell because it is easier to understand and measure.

You can conveniently divide performance into three dimensions: clinical, service, and financial. While these are interdependent and in aggregate define system performance, for clarity and for strategy development it is a useful distinction. Certain groups will tend to focus on one area and need to understand the interrelationship of all three. Physicians will typically focus on traditional clinical outcomes such as mortality or procedural complications and will be less likely to be aware of resource consumption, length of stay, or patient satisfaction scores. Nurses may tend to focus on skill outcomes, medication errors, or patient complaint measures and be unaware of long-term survival outcomes. Private or staff clinic nurses may have no access to performance measures and no mechanism to implement them. Clinic managers may know the volume of phone calls, average wait time, or number of visits per physician but may have no knowledge of patient volume by diagnosis, cost per encounter, or immunization rate for clinic patients.

In actuality, there is a universe of measurable items that can reflect performance in all three areas. The challenge is to develop a manageable set of valid and reliable measures to use as performance indicators and then to have a strategy for using those measures to promote improvement effectively. The typical mistakes are to measure too much and to present the measures in isolation—in both time and topic. To be truly useful, performance measures must be shown in relationship to each other and cast as trends over time. An integrated system must be able to apply performance measures across the span of care and service sites.

If the measures selected are valid, the most effective way to use them for improving performance is to share them in appropriate settings in a nonthreatening and constructive manner. They must be presented in context of overall performance, and successes should be widely shared and celebrated. It is particularly useful to present aggregate clinical discipline or program measures to entire interdisciplinary work teams. If all members of a team, whatever size, have knowledge of their performance, they will by their very nature want to improve. If a culture is imbued with a clear understanding of the organization's vision, mission, and goals, and people have valid measures of their performance, improvement will become an everyday attitude. This for me was best said by Aristotle: "We are what we continually do. Excellence, therefore, is not an act but a habit."

Physician Integration and Leadership

The importance of the role of physicians in clinical integration cannot be overemphasized. The more that practicing physicians, whether in private practice, academic appointment, or a staff model system, play an integral role in the governance and operations of a delivery system, the more successful the organization. Physician leaders must be chosen with care and for the right reasons. The most effective physician leaders are those who are respected by their peers as clinicians, who understand and share the values of the organization, who support its mission, and who live the concepts of collaborative practice and team effort. This does not mean that they are full-time vice president or senior management–level employees, although they may be. Some systems have found that employing system-level vice presidents for medical affairs is an effective strategy for promoting system-level clinical integration. However, many of the most effective leaders can and will remain in private clinical practice and have the ability to balance occasional conflicting interests.

Physician participation should be considered at all levels of the delivery system, from corporate board to local clinic or operating unit. Some of the most innovative and rapidly evolving systems have explicit strategies to maximize physician presence on their boards of directors, including chair positions. Others have plans, including budgets for physician-leader development, to encourage participation at operating units or on systemwide councils. Significant opportunities for physician leadership revolve around new and innovative medical staff structures that transcend traditional departmental models in favor of interdisciplinary disease management teams or clinically focused programs. These can be organized around a disease population, such as diabetics or asthmatics, or around a functionally related set, such as maternal and child care, cardiovascular services, or neurosciences.

Physician involvement at the levels noted will require significant time and resource commitments. In addition to the leadership positions just described, there are myriad opportunities for productive physician involvement in interdisciplinary clinical and operational initiatives that should be actively encouraged. Barriers to participation, including time commitment, accountability, and compensation, should be dealt with in a forthright manner.

The efforts of a large, rapidly evolving delivery system in the Midwest illustrates the commitment to physician leadership and integration. The board of directors of this corporation is chaired by a practicing physician. Physicians in clinical practice either chair or are members of every board committee. Similarly, practicing physicians are on the boards of every hospital within the system. A systemwide physician advisory council has direct reporting and advisory access to the corporate board. There are vice presidents for medical affairs at urban and rural regional hospitals—all physicians in full-time appointments. Systemwide clinical best practices interdisciplinary teams organized around high-priority disease states are led by paid medical directors, all of whom are in private clinical practice. The best practices teams are charged with recommending to senior management strategies for best clinical practices dissemination, resource commitment, information system resource needs, and outcome measurements across the entire continuum of care for that disease condition. Within the system, two hospital medical staffs have combined, eliminating traditional departments in favor of interdisciplinary teams. Practicing physicians are employed part-time at each site as chief of staff and clinical coordinators for medicine and surgery, paid with combined hospital and medical staff funds. Several clinical disease management programs have practicing physicians as medical advisers on a contractual basis. The charge and accountability of physicians at each level of clinical activity is to maximize interdisciplinary and collaborative practice and to integrate activities across the inpatient-outpatient spectrum.

Conclusion

Based on my experience in clinical practice and in my other roles, clinical integration is the logical expression of best practices. It demands of us the best effort and highest standards that our profession calls for: to wherever possible prevent disease, to heal the sick, and to comfort the dying. It asks that we attend to the needs of our communities and that we be wise stewards of resources—basing our decisions and our work on shared values and measured outcomes. Because there are many who participate in improving the health of a community, we must work together toward carefully defined goals that are within the scope of our ability. It requires a willingness to promote and manage change and to be advocates for those we serve. The foundations of success in this endeavor will always be the culture of the organizations we work in and our desire to continually improve our performance.

Chapter Four

Applying Systems Thinking
to Clinical Integration

Ann Scott Blouin, Jonathan Kaplan, Barbara Buturusis

Chapter Three describes the essential role of values and culture in clinical integration. This chapter outlines a systems approach to integrating the components and elements of a health care enterprise.

Health care enterprises are investigating creative strategies to integrate and organize their services in response to the relentless demands of managed care. Although motivations vary, they are usually driven by the need to survive today's chaotic health care environment.

In this environment, governmental and nongovernmental payers are putting unprecedented pressure on organizations to reduce costs, while consumers and accrediting agencies (along with payers) are demanding improved performance. In response, providers have formed affiliations or acquired new partners in an effort to survive and thrive in this rapidly changing, aggressive health care marketplace.

The key to success is the ability to successfully integrate clinical and administrative capabilities across the affiliating organizations to create a new, successful enterprise. These organizations and the resulting new enterprise benefit from a systems approach for planning and decision making.

Defining the Enterprise

An *enterprise*, for the purposes of this chapter, is defined as those components and elements that come together from the affiliating organizations to provide an infrastructure for the delivery of health care services. Enterprise *components* include clinical, educational, and research entities. *Elements* represent strategic and operational structures and processes within the enterprise.

Components

The *clinical component* refers to the delivery of health care services across the continuum of care. These entities include everything from prevention and wellness programs to hospice care, delivered everywhere from the patient's home to the intensive care unit. The *educational component* varies by type of organization or enterprise. It includes medical, nursing, or allied health schools and their management. If the enterprise has a *research component*, its programs may include clinical (applied) research, bench research, grant management, and population-based research.

Elements

The *operational elements* include support functions such as materials management, food and nutrition, maintenance, diagnostic testing, and ancillary support. These elements exist to support the clinical component and are crucial to the efficient delivery of health care services.

The *strategic elements* include structures that are key to the development and performance of the enterprise and are often centralized. The key strategic elements include the board or executive governing body and the functions of human resources, provider relations, payer contracting, public relations, finance, quality, information systems, purchasing, and governmental relations.

The evolution and success of the enterprise depends on the effective integration of these components and elements among all of the organizations that it encompasses. In order to ensure integration, a systems approach to critical success factors and enterprise capabilities is essential.

Critical Success Factors

Enterprises must analyze their critical success factors. Nine of these critical success factors are outlined in this section.

1. Clear Goals, Strategic Direction, and Aligned Incentives

The organizations must define what the new enterprise is or will be. Organizations must clarify the new mission, values, vision, and culture to ensure that all the organizational components are moving in a common direction, aligned with the priorities of the enterprise. Several provocative questions can stimulate dialogue about strategic direction:

- What are the reasons for integration? Are they purely financial, or is there a motivation to deliver coordinated care across the continuum to a larger number of patients?
- Which model of integration will position the enterprise for success? Which partnerships are key and offer the greatest level of integration with the greatest efficiency and economy of scale? Are the incentives aligned for key constituencies?
- How will enterprise members preserve and expand market share? Have they identified partners with the qualities required to deliver increased volume and market presence?

2. Improved Financial Outcomes

Increased efficiencies will be required for future success. The coordinated use of capital assets will assist in achieving enterprise financial goals. The enterprise must maximize its competitive advantage by reducing operating costs through achieving economies of scale, increasing purchasing power, and integrating clinical and financial data to support decision making. Critical financial indicators must be monitored closely for trends that may signal success or adverse performance.

The enterprise must specifically address financial issues such as the following:

- How will the enterprise manage finances, including the accountability and distribution methods for both positive and negative financial results?
- How will the enterprise merge financial and clinical success factors so that decision making and prioritization of resource allocation ensures clinical quality and financial success?

3. Strong Physician Partnerships

Enterprises should strive to create opportunities for maximum clinical and economic integration with physician partners. It is important to consider how financial and nonfinancial incentives for physicians will be addressed and aligned in the integrated system (see Chapter Six). Joint contracting by the organizations and physicians with payers can be valuable in aligning incentives in the areas of quality, utilization, and cost.

4. Wider Geographic Coverage

Broadening the provision of services over a wider geographic region is necessary to be attractive to payers, provide convenience to patients, and capture new market share. The combined geography of partner organizations can significantly expand the opportunities for volume and revenue. Integrating and coordinating enterprise initiatives across this geography is a high priority.

5. Effective Medical Management Functions

Medical management functions maximize the clinical component through management of care, utilization, and demand. The enterprise must address how medical management functions and their relationship to payer contracting will be integrated across the enterprise.

Medical management is of strategic importance and is made up of activities designed to reduce the overall requirement for health care services (Kongstvedt, 1996). For example, Plocher (Kongstvedt, 1996) has identified five different types of demand management activities: (1) nurse advice lines, (2) self-care and medical consumerism programs, (3) shared decision-making programs, (4) medical informatics, and (5) preventive services and health risk appraisal.

6. Improved Payer Partnerships

The development of partnerships with payers is critical to capturing managed care volume. When physicians and the enterprise contract jointly, such as with contract management organization (CMO) structures, they present a unified presence to payers. Enterprise contracting capability and skill in managing risk will be strengthened through strong physician-payer partnerships.

7. Integrated Information Systems

Information systems that integrate clinical and financial information for individual providers and the enterprise are critical. Creating linkages among registration, clinical documentation, coding, and billing and collections functions will be invaluable in optimizing revenue flow and clinical efficiency. For example, if demographic and insurance information were transferred in real time among all departments, bills could be processed with fewer errors, which would reduce days in accounts receivable and improve cash collections. In addition, patients would not have to provide the same information at each point of service, thus improving patient satisfaction. A further improvement occurs with the seamless electronic transfer of account information between provider and payer. In our experience, the single most significant obstacle to integration of an enterprise, besides culture, is the lack of integrated information systems.

8. Centralization and Decentralization Criteria

A clear set of criteria for centralization and decentralization of enterprise components and elements provides structure for achieving coordinated decision making and economies of scale.

Decentralized functions are usually site-specific and relate to technical delivery of services or products. In our experience, there may be enterprise standards, but delivery and first-line management of service are decentralized. These services include clinical care delivery (on patient care units, respiratory therapy, point-of-care testing, and so on) and financial counseling (customized to the patient's situation).

Functions that are usually *centralized* or shared assist in executing enterprise strategy and achieving integration. These include

- *Governance:* board and executive staff composition, physician governance, collective bargaining activities
- *Strategic planning:* market assessment, public relations, contracting, enterprise development and integration strategies, community relationships, master site planning, and facility development
- *Medical staff functions:* credentialing, recruitment, medical education, and research funding
- *Financial management:* revenue cycle, optimization of reimbursement, investment management, capital funding
- *Contracting:* with payers for services and with suppliers for group purchasing

A centralization-decentralization matrix that outlines key elements and decision criteria will aid in decision making and identify the option that delivers the greatest value to the enterprise and its patients.

9. Coordinated Care Delivery to Achieve Clinical Outcomes

Horizontal integration can ensure consistency in care access. For example, a multihospital system may implement system-level CareMaps (where care is provided to congestive heart failure patients in the same timetable and with the same goals). Enterprise success may rest in the ability to influence rather than own all care provided to a patient. This is especially true if the enterprise has assumed risk for payment but cannot afford to own every point on the continuum of care. The ability to influence all points along the continuum is key to controlling clinical outcomes and managing financial risk. Forming effective partnerships with other provider organizations is therefore as essential as skillful partnering with physicians and payers.

In his book *The Death of Competition*, Moore (1996) stated that competition, as most of us have known it, is dead. Any business that does not recognize this fact is threatened. The need for direct head-to-head competition is diminishing, while the need for "co-evolution" is intensifying. Moore asserted that even "excellent businesses can be destroyed by the conditions around them" (p. 5). Creating new markets requires that competitors cooperate, not compete, to create a workable economic future—generating shared visions, forming alliances, and managing complex relationships.

Core Processes

The core processes of a health care enterprise are ensuring patient access and securing market share; delivering care and services; and demonstrating outcomes. Because these core processes are interrelated and are critical to the success of the enterprise, a systems approach is best used. As the enterprise makes decisions and prioritizes allocation of system resources, it should not compromise the delicate balance between these core processes. Figure 4.1 illustrates the interrelationship and flow among these processes as the organization manages its future.

Ensuring Access and Securing the Market

An enterprise must understand the market it serves and the one it wishes to serve. An assessment of the marketplace and a coordinated marketing strategy will ensure that the proper services are developed and that strategic partnering with appropriate alliances strengthens the enterprise. Knowledge of risks and opportunities is essential for informed decision making. Strategies for securing a market include mergers and acquisitions; community outreach and education; managed care contracting; and accepting and managing risk.

Delivering Care and Services

Potential benefits of integration include opportunities to enter new markets, build a continuum of care in existing markets, and implement systemwide care protocols or clinical paths to ensure best practices (see Chapter Eight). When assessing current care delivery methodologies and anticipating future ones, consideration must

Figure 4.1. Managing Core Processes of the Enterprise.

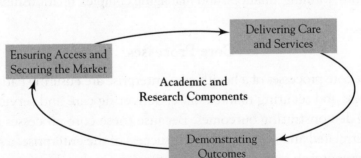

be given to access and distribution channels, clinical integration, and capacity management.

Access and Distribution Channels. What does the enterprise bring to the market relative to the continuum of care? Which of the following services does it own and which can it effectively influence and coevolve?

- Preventive care
- Primary and ambulatory care
- Specialty and ambulatory care centers
- Acute ambulatory care (ambulatory surgery centers, urgent care centers, day hospitals, infusion suites)
- Acute inpatient care
- Tertiary and referral
- Regional care
- Home health care
- Subacute care
- Alternative medicine
- Long-term care
- Assisted and transitional living
- Hospice care

Care Delivery. The key to success for care delivery is coordination across the continuum. Capabilities must include education and wellness planning and disease and care management. It is no longer appropriate to populate an enterprise with clinical paths that address only hospital admission to discharge. A holistic continuum approach is required to achieve the best outcomes in the most efficient manner. The enterprise must be able to address the following areas with expertise:

- Health risk appraisal
- Care planning
- Information management and documentation
- Ancillary management (internal or external ancillaries, shared or regional services)
- Patient compliance management
- Pharmacy and drug management

Capacity Management. The integrated enterprise must be attentive to the use of its resources. It is no longer sufficient simply to monitor clinical personnel numbers as a financial strategy. Instead, to ensure desired outcomes the enterprise must monitor a broader range of indicators:

- Management and efficient deployment of all resources (capital funds, operational funds, marketing and public relations capacity)
- Maximization of intellectual capital (valuing and using human talent and creativity to gain a competitive advantage)
- Resource scheduling management (efficient scheduling of providers with varying volumes, diagnostic equipment, operating rooms, and so on)
- Facilities and plant efficiencies (proper allocation of square footage, master facility development plan, and so on)

Demonstrating Outcomes

The development of processes to measure clinical outcomes and costs and to produce provider profiles are essential. The ability to track clinical and financial outcomes is useful for demonstrating value to employees and payers and identifying the positive or negative path of the enterprise. Accurate and timely information and vigilance in managing successful cost and quality outcomes are essential.

Cost, Quality, and Service Strategies. The delicate interrelationships among cost, quality, and service necessitate a continuous quality improvement program that uses a systems approach. Such an approach integrates clinical standards, accreditation standards, licensing requirements, and customer satisfaction with administrative priorities, including cost and quality management.

Value to Constituencies. A well-integrated enterprise can deliver added value to its constituencies as follows:

- *To patients and the community:* the enterprise can provide clinical care that demonstrates focus on wellness, prevention, improved outcomes, and cost-effectiveness in addressing the health care needs of the community it serves.
- *To the board and executive management:* outcomes should move the organization toward meeting its mission and delivering the strategic benefits of promoting financial viability, increased market share, and resources for recapitalization.
- *To management and staff:* an enterprise that values its people attends to job satisfaction and alignment of individual and organizational rewards and incentives. The opportunities for career development and greater job security due to the growth of the enterprise and increasing enlargement or sophistication of current jobs can serve as a retention strategy for talented staff within the system.

Integrated Health Care Delivery Systems

Peter Senge, a systems thinking expert, describes a business as a system "bound by invisible fabrics of interrelated actions, which often take years to fully play out their effects on each other" (1990, p. 7). He noted that businesses tend to focus on moments in time, or snapshots of parts of the system, instead of the whole. Senge calls for a new approach to management known as *systems thinking,* which he defines as "a conceptual framework . . . to make the full patterns clearer and to see how to change them effectively" (p. 7).

Integrated health care delivery systems, perhaps more than any other type of enterprise, require systems thinking. The enterprise is made up of components and elements, and the relationships between them define its structure. The clinical and financial relationships between the components and elements of the enterprise are created by its mission and the patients that move across the enterprise. In order to maximize integration, the enterprise must be conceptualized and managed as a system. Systems theory can provide a framework for this endeavor.

Systems Archetypes

Archetypes are valuable tools for seeing issues from a systems thinking perspective (Senge, 1990; Kim, 1993). *Systems archetypes* are common systems structures that can serve various purposes:

- As a "lens" through which the enterprise can view a compelling question or complex initiative
- As a pattern or template for diagnosing a complicated issue or problem
- As a theory to structure discussion
- As a tool for predicting behavior

Archetypes can also stimulate provocative questions and help anticipate the effect of change on the performance of the enterprise.

While archetypes can be used in myriad ways, for the purpose of our case study the "drifting goals" archetype has been selected as a theory to structure discussion. In this archetype, the gap between the current reality and the desired future state is resolved through one of two actions: the enterprise can take a selected action to reach the future state or it can lower the expectation of the desired future state. The predisposition of an enterprise under pressure is to address problems, particularly if they are financial in nature, by lowering its future expectation. Over time, continually lowering goals erodes the quality of clinical and financial performance. The case study presented later in the chapter will describe two organizations that merge to create an integrated delivery network. The archetype will analyze their approach to integration by using a systems thinking framework.

Critical Assessments and Decisions

Integration of clinical and administrative concerns is the key to success of the enterprise; the level of integration that has been achieved must be reassessed periodically as a guide to further planning and decision making. As a first step in the process of assessment, the current state must be defined. This requires a review of external and internal market factors. *External market factors* and capabilities that are likely to have an impact on integration include

- Competitor analysis
- Community needs assessment
- Payer analysis
- Legal and regulatory review

Internal factors that are likely to have an impact on integration include

- Organizational structure and infrastructure
- Medical staff management
- Financial management
- Communication
- Incentives and compensation
- Quality initiatives and outcomes
- Information management

- Risk management
- Patient, provider, and staff satisfaction

Having established the internal and external factors, the *desired future state* must then be defined. As part of this process, enablers and barriers need to be identified and addressed. The enterprise must develop a collective purpose and vision, confirm values, and identify key success factors. The ability to implement change in bridging gaps between the current and future state will determine success.

Case Study

An academic medical center and a community hospital have decided to pursue an affiliation that is intended to create an integrated delivery system. Their business goals are to capture market share and improve financial performance by bringing together complementary services and programs.

Current State Assessment and Future State Design

The academic medical center brings capabilities in tertiary care, with concomitant research and educational processes. The community hospital brings capabilities in community outreach and primary, rehabilitative, and subacute care. The current state capabilities of the combined organizations are evaluated using a capabilities table tool that contains the categories included in Table 4.1.

The capabilities table lists four tiers that the enterprise uses to rate its current state. Each tier represents a coevolution toward the desired state. The current capabilities are compared to the desired state of the enterprise, represented by the fourth tier on the table.

The current-state information is then plotted on a "spider" diagram, in which the outer perimeter represents the desired future state (see Figure 4.2). The spider diagram presents a visual tool for assessing enterprise integration and identifying gaps in the desired

Table 4.1. Capabilities Table.

Capability	Tier One	Tier Two	Tier Three	Tier Four
Goals, Vision, and Strategic Direction	Goals are unclear, the organization lacks a vision for the future state. There is little or no planning.	Goals are being defined but do not relate to critical success factors for integration. The vision is not well articulated.	Goals are clear. The vision has been developed and is in the early phase of communication.	Goals are clear and documented. The vision is clear, and staff are able to articulate it. The vision and goals reflect integration.
Motivation and Incentives	Not addressed.	Discussions about motivation and incentives are taking place.	Motivation and incentives are being aligned with the enterprise priorities.	Motivation and incentives are aligned with the organizational priority for integration.
Systems Approach	Components and elements of the enterprise are addressed in a parallel, unrelated manner. Shifting the burden is occurring in each organization.	Components and elements of the enterprise are considered to be related. Decision making and planning are conducted in parallel fashion.	Components and elements are partially integrated. Initiatives are seen as having system effects.	Components and elements are fully integrated. Initiatives are viewed through the lens of archetypes.
Core Processes	Core processes are not recognized nor addressed in any substantive manner.	Core processes are recognized, but no integrated efforts are planned.	Core processes are recognized and are the focus of integration efforts.	Core processes are viewed in the context of components and elements. Efforts address the entire enterprise.

Table 4.1. Capabilities Table. (*continued*)

Capability	Tier One	Tier Two	Tier Three	Tier Four
Centralization and Decentralization	Centralization and decentralization are arbitrary. No criteria are identified.	Centralization and decentralization are based on instincts. No analysis is done.	Centralization and decentralization are based on criteria. Modeling and analysis are not completed.	Centralization and decentralization are based on criteria. Modeling and analysis are completed.
Payer Partnerships	Managed care contracts are limited. Payers view the organization as nonresponsive.	Managed care contracts are in place. No payer partnership is identified. Satisfaction with services and costs is low.	Active and ongoing negotiations are occurring. Satisfaction with services and costs are moderate.	Payers identify the integrated system as one entity. Satisfaction with services and costs is high.
Value Added to Constituencies	Constituencies view the organization as ineffective and unresponsive.	The board views the organization as taking the proper business direction. The community and employees are dissatisfied with the system.	The board and the community view the enterprise as having business acumen and adding value to the health of the community. Staff satisfaction is improving.	All constituencies view the integrated organization as adding value to the health of the community and the satisfaction of the staff.

Table 4.1. Capabilities Table. (*continued*)

Capability	Tier One	Tier Two	Tier Three	Tier Four
Care Delivery and Clinical Outcomes	Care delivery is not protocol-driven. Outcomes are not measured. Patient satisfaction is low.	Few clinical paths are developed for inpatient care. Patient satisfaction is moderate.	Clinical paths are comprehensive. Outcomes are being measured. Patient satisfaction is good.	Clinical paths guide the provision of care across the enterprise. Outcomes are measured and reported. Patient satisfaction is high.
Financial Outcomes	The enterprise is demonstrating serious financial losses, and the trend is downward. Capital funds are limited. Labor cost reductions are necessary and based on a dollar requirement.	The enterprise is experiencing financial losses, but the trend is improving. Labor reductions are necessary and based on a dollar requirement.	The enterprise is generating a margin. Funds are available for capital purchases. Labor reductions are necessary, but a systems process is applied.	The enterprise is generating a strong financial picture. New programs can be funded. The organization is demonstrating growth.
Information Systems	Information systems are not integrated. They do not support clinical advancements or financial integration. Hardware is outdated.	Information systems are not integrated. They do not support clinical advancements and have limited value for the revenue cycle. Hardware is outdated.	Information systems are being upgraded with a focus on clinical and financial integration. Hardware is being upgraded.	Information systems have been upgraded, with a focus on clinical and financial integration. Hardware is upgraded, and implementation is proceeding.

Table 4.1. Capabilities Table. (*continued*)

Capability	Tier One	Tier Two	Tier Three	Tier Four
Physician Partnerships	Physicians exhibit no commitment to the enterprise. Relationships are counterproductive.	Physicians exhibit limited commitment to the enterprise.	Physicians jointly contract with the enterprise.	Physicians provide leadership to the enterprise and view their success as linked to that of the enterprise.
Medical Management	Medical management functions do not exist and are not being planned.	Medical management functions are being considered.	Medical management is planned or partially implemented.	Medical management is developed and operational.
Geography	The organizations have overlapping service areas. No gain in market share or coverage is anticipated.	The organizations have some overlapping service areas. A small gain in market share or coverage is possible.	The organizations have minimal overlapping service areas. A moderate gain in market share is possible.	The organizations have complimentary service areas. A significant gain in market share is possible.

Figure 4.2. Case Study Spider Diagram: Clinical and Administrative Integration Capacity.

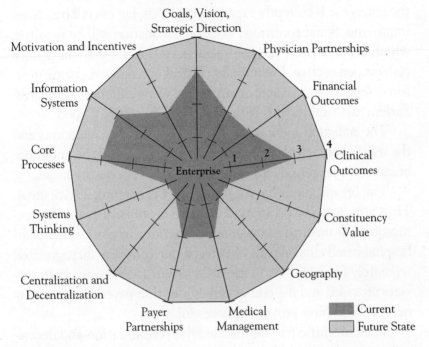

future state. It also facilitates the use of a systems thinking approach, as mapping the capabilities interdependently creates a picture of the whole enterprise.

The spider diagram can suggest priorities in closing the gap between the current and future states. It also assists in identifying competing initiatives and parallel processes that may compromise the integration initiative.

The enterprise is depicted in the center of the spider diagram in Figure 4.2. The current capabilities, as listed in the capabilities table, are ranked. In this case, the goals, vision, clinical outcomes, core processes, and information systems that the enterprise has developed are their strongest capabilities. However, the enterprise is in the early phase of documenting and communicating these to the larger organization.

Physicians are skeptical about the entire enterprise. They have not exhibited commitment to the strategic direction. Financially, the enterprise is currently experiencing losses, but overall trends are improving. Some continued workforce reduction will be required, which unfortunately has been addressed thus far without using a systems perspective. Preliminary clinical outcomes are being measured separately by each organization using different standards. Patient satisfaction with clinical services, however, is good.

The affiliation and its rationale has confused the community and the staff. There is little commitment to the success of the enterprise because of a perceived lack of added value to key constituencies.

The organizations have significantly overlapping service areas. Thus anticipated gain in market share is unlikely. Neither organization has medical management functions in place other than hospital-based clinical paths. Managed care contracts are negotiated separately for each organization. Payer satisfaction with both services provided and the cost of care is low; thus payer-provider partnering efforts have proven unsuccessful.

The enterprise has approached the centralization and decentralization of services in an arbitrary manner. There are no defined criteria, and management is confused about the direction and rationale for changing organizational structures.

Core processes are the focus of improvement efforts at each organization but are not integrated. Care delivery systems remain separate and, in many cases, redundant, without economies of scale available with integrated care management across the continuum.

Information systems are being upgraded. There is a plan to integrate them across the enterprise and between clinical and administrative functions. A plan for hardware upgrade has been funded.

Discussions about aligning incentives are taking place, but action has not been taken. This has led to skepticism by key constituencies, especially physicians. The enterprise has failed to address alignment of incentives and appears to accept the lack of progress.

On balance, the enterprise is not using a systems approach. Enterprise components and elements continue to be addressed in a parallel and unrelated manner by each organization. Although the goals and strategic direction are clear, the organizations continue to act as separate entities with separate clinical and administrative functions. The organizations may be allowing their initial goals to drift and are rationalizing not moving toward implementing the benefits of the future state because of difficulty in obtaining buy-in from key constituencies. The organization, as reflected by their executive leadership, yield to the pressure and accept a lower level of integration than originally intended.

Drifting Goals

In the case study, as the enterprise moves toward bridging the gap, managers need to be aware of drifting goals. For example, in achieving the desired financial outcomes, the workforce is reduced without a systems analysis. The enterprise convinces itself that it must reduce full-time employees (FTE) to generate an improved financial picture without analyzing the effect on clinical outcomes, constituency support, and payer relationships. Without a systems approach analysis, deterioration can occur in other capabilities. This is especially true if the FTE calculations are based only on the individual entity's necessary dollar reduction in cost and not on core process improvement. A systems thinking framework, applied to all components and elements of the enterprise and its entities, can minimize adverse clinical and financial risk.

Closing the Gap Through Reengineering

In review, the spider diagram inner graph represents the current state of the enterprise. The outer perimeter represents the ideal, future state. Tier four of the capabilities table describes the ideal state. The gap for each capability is the difference between the current and ideal state. The organization can use this information to devise an action plan for each capability to achieve the future state. They can also use the diagram to identify drifting goals or situations where they have lowered the goal from the ideal state due to factors in their current reality.

Here is an example of a how a systems-thinking organization successfully used systems thinking as referenced by the spider diagram to improve its clinical and functional integration. The enterprise set its goals at the fourth level of the capabilities table, in partnership with key constituencies (such as the community, physicians, payers, and staff). Leadership educated the partners on the business imperative for the ideal state and the risk of drifting goals. Further, leadership used the capabilities table and spider diagram to monitor for behaviors that potentially lowered their goals in response to organization pressure. In using the tool and the consensus that had been gained toward the desired state, they stayed focused on the outcome and prevented the integration from being less than optimal.

Conclusion

The successful health care delivery enterprise will define itself carefully and understand its elements and components. The new enterprise will identify and monitor success factors that are critical to creating a bridge from the current to future state. It will demonstrate a systems approach to planning and action that will ensure that the clinical and administrative integration goal is not lowered due to current pressures. Yielding to pressure in lowering the goal can cause decreasing performance over time, suboptimal realization of integration benefits, and, eventually, the failure of the enterprise.

Using systems thinking can be a rewarding and productive method to integrating clinical, educational, and research components of emerging integrated health care delivery systems.

References

Kim, D. H. (1993). Drifting goals: The "boiled frog" syndrome. In *Systems archetypes I: Diagnosing systemic issues and designing high leverage interventions* (pp. 11–12). Boston: Pegasus Communications.

Kongstvedt, P. (1996). Managing medical-surgical utilization. In Kongstvedt, P. (Ed.), *The managed health care handbook* (pp. 249–251). Gaithersburg, MD: Aspen Publishers.

Moore, J. F. (1996). *The death of competition: Leadership and strategy in the age of ecosystems.* New York: HarperBusiness.

Senge, P. M. (1990). *The fifth discipline: The art and practice of the learning organization.* New York: Doubleday Currency.

Chapter Five

Administrative Integration Through Product and Service Line Structure

Sharon A. Henry

As Chapter Four described, enterprisewide reengineering can be a strategy for administrative or clinical integration. This chapter focuses specifically on administrative integration.

Product or service line organization is a powerful approach to creating an integrated administrative infrastructure to support clinical integration. Organizing around product lines facilitates clinical integration by focusing the clinical and administrative team's attention on meeting patient needs across a broader continuum of care. This chapter describes a 1990s version of clinical product line organization within a larger IDS.

A Short History of Product Line Organization

Many early attempts to establish service or product lines had a marketing focus. In this type of product line structure, an organization identified *products*, or programs that it wished to sell, and organized around them. Because this approach had an external marketing focus rather than a patient-centered focus, it provided little support for collaborative practice. Moreover, it was common for each program to organize and manage itself as a separate "silo" within the overall organization. These separate silos were frequently unconnected to the organization as a whole and developed costly, redundant services to support their operations. In summary, these early, marketing-focused product line structures failed to successfully address critical issues such as outcomes management, resource stewardship, quality improvement, and collaborative relationships. Consequently, many such models were abandoned because goals were not met or vision was redirected. Functional organizations (such as departments of nursing, pharmacy, and so on) often replaced the obsolete product line structures. However, this model also failed to address program needs and facilitate disease management.

Managed care and capitation have led to a renewed interest in product line organization as a strategy to support the management of specific patient populations across sites and over time. Some organizations have established product lines that are clearly connected to the larger organization but have also left traditional management structures in place. For example, there may be strong product lines that are not profit-and-loss centers. Instead, the traditional entities—hospitals and their departments—retain budgetary authority, and the product lines coexist. A smaller number of organizations have implemented product line management in the place of traditional management structures. Budgetary responsibility is transferred to the product lines, and they replace the previous organizational structure. Finally, there are some organizations with leaders who believe that the product line concept is artificial and not particularly helpful, and they have no interest in it.

The product line structure presented in this chapter organizes and manages a clinical program for the care of cardiovascular patients, with full profit-and-loss responsibility. The experience described here demonstrates that this type of product line structure can improve both business and clinical outcomes.

Clinical Product Lines

A *clinical product line* is generally described by the types of cases or disease entities on which it focuses, as well as the outpatient programs and services associated with provision of care. For example, the cardiovascular product line at the Mercy and Unity Hospitals of Minnesota's Allina Health system encompasses all inpatient, outpatient, diagnostic, interventional, rehabilitative, and preventive services and programs for patients in case types described in DRGs 102 through 145. The product line structure is designed to directly or indirectly organize, develop, and manage all aspects of the service line and to be accountable for all of the outcomes, both qualitative and quantitative, for the customers served.

As operations director for this product line and program, I provide management direction to staff in order to meet the administrative, clinical, and service needs of both inpatients and ambulatory patients. Specific accountabilities include (1) planning and implementing programs to address product line, hospital, and system goals; (2) providing operational leadership within the service line; (3) selecting and developing a management team; (4) designing a collaborative model with the medical staff and all service line interfaces; and (5) negotiating budgets and managing the financial performance for the entire product line. The organizational structure is depicted in Figure 5.1.

Key success factors for this kind of organization include a partnership between the medical director and operations director, progressive medical staff leadership within the hospital program, support from senior management, and committed staff. These elements must then converge to create a visionary team.

Goal-Directed Management

The outcomes of any organizational structure must, of course, meet the goals of the larger system. I have watched those goals change dramatically over the past thirty years in health care. *Value* is the key word being touted now by most providers and payers as they seek their share of the available market; but what does *value* translate to in the real world of care delivery? It must translate to program goals that meet the strategic goals of the organization, the operational goals of the providers, the fiscal restraints of the marketplace, and the expectations of those receiving services.

Figure 5.1. Mercy and Unity Hospitals' Allina Health System Organizational Chart.

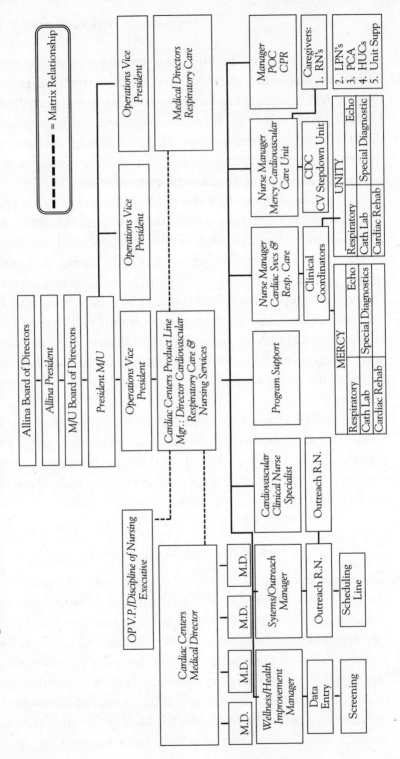

We must articulate all of these goals clearly to gain commitment from those who implement them. They must be measurable to evaluate outcomes of care and service on all levels. The best place to articulate the goals of a product line or program is the yearly business plan.

Organizational goals should be formulated on several levels, from the larger organization to the specific work plans of each individual team. I am periodically asked to provide consultation to other organizations, and, in that capacity, I have observed organizations in which business plans are developed by one executive, distributed annually, and collect dust on a high shelf for the remainder of the year. Business plans must be living documents, developed collaboratively by the entire team and used continually to improve processes on the journey toward goal achievement. Examples of strategic goals that drill down to individual work plans and measurement criteria are outlined in the next section.

Strategic Goals Link Systems, Hospitals, and Programs

Allina is an IDS that includes a health plan, acute care hospitals, physician providers, home care, long-term care, transportation, and other diversified health services. Located in Minnesota, Allina is a major provider and plan in a heavily managed care market.

The following examples illustrate the overall vision of the health system, with the stated cardiovascular mission of the integrated hospitals supporting the vision and drilling down to the individual hospital and program goals.

> *The Allina vision:* Allina will be the recognized innovator in community health improvement.
>
> *The Allina mission:* to provide an excellent health care experience for our customers.
>
> *The Allina values:* service, innovation, partnership, integrity, and stewardship.

The Allina Cardiovascular Steering Team mission supports the Allina vision by pursuing recognition as an innovator in the improvement of cardiovascular health for the communities that we serve. Further, Allina's cardiovascular (CV) services are committed to creating an enhanced cardiac delivery system that achieves the following goals:

- Delivers care through easily accessible and coordinated services provided in the most effective manner
- Achieves quality outcomes that improve the health and well-being of our patients
- Provides the highest level of treatment through early application of breakthrough technology and active involvement in clinical research
- Partners with other Allina providers to develop a broad geographical delivery system
- Provides integrated, consistent care based on advanced practice protocols, which are shared and implemented throughout the system
- Develops and maintains a superb education program for health care professionals
- Creates value through the appropriate and efficient utilization of resources
- Improves the health of people living in the communities we serve

The Allina Cardiovascular Steering Team's three-year goal is to consciously pursue opportunities for delivering appropriate, effective, and efficient care and to add value to our services. An infrastructure of vision, mission, goals, and objectives moves from one level to the next in a pyramid structure in successful organizations. All programs and services support the next level with clear understanding and solid transitions up and down the structure.

Moving from the collective cardiovascular services of all the system's hospitals to an individual hospital is the next step.

Mercy and Unity Hospitals' vision is the Allina shared vision. Mercy and Unity Hospitals strive to further the Allina shared mission by meeting the following goals:

- Providing high-quality and cost-effective inpatient, outpatient, and long-term care
- Collaborating with others to improve the health of the communities we serve

Resource stewardship is a three-year goal for the hospitals that necessitates continued improvement in its cost structure to respond to market demands for value in both quality and cost. For Mercy and Unity Hospitals' Cardiac Program, resource stewardship means continuous quality improvement to (1) coordinate, refine, and expand operational aspects of the Cardiac Centers and (2) provide customer groups with improved outcomes, lower costs, and maximum access and satisfaction, as the excerpt from the program business plan in Table 5.1 shows.

These goals are measured as follows:

- Financial goals are measured by contribution margin and attainment of cost reduction targets.
- Business goals are measured by market share.
- Clinical quality improvement goals are measured by achievement of stated quality indicators.
- Customer expectation goals are measured by service quality polls of patients/families, payers, and physicians.
- Process goals are measured with well-documented improvements in targeted processes, achieved by continuously engaging providers in the plan, do, study, act (PDSA cycle) CQI methodology.

Table 5.1. Cardiac Centers 1997: Cardiology Goals, Objectives, and Strategies.

Objectives	Strategies	Priority	Time Frame	Responsible Person
1a. To motivate and empower professional staff to evaluate and improve care delivery systems and further refine care management for our patients and families.	a. Continued refinement and improvement of concurrent case management systems (including clinical pathways/CareMaps). Goal: ALOS ↓, improved outcomes, ↓ cost, increased profit margin, and continuously improved quality of care. Develop action plans to address identified areas of improvement from variance analysis.	1	1998–Ongoing 1998–Ongoing	Administration, Program Director, Medical Director, Systems Manager, Unit Nursing Directors, Nurse Managers, Staff Nurses, CV C.A.T. Teams, Cardiology, CV Surgeons, CV Work Team, Finance, and Quality/Case Management and Peer Review Team.
1b/c. Evaluate cardiovascular program and product line quarterly.	b. Quarterly analysis of all available data to evaluate programs in relation to our competitors in the marketplace. • Develop work plans to deal with identified areas for systems and process improvement based on data analysis.	1	1998–1999 1998–1999	→
	c. Physician-specific data presented to individual groups "blinded" in peer review meetings.	1	1998	→
1d. Development of best practice guidelines and	d. Best practice model • Acute MI Guidelines • Angina; chest pain evaluation units	1	1998–Ongoing 1998–Ongoing 1998–Ongoing	→ →

	Action	Timeline		Responsibility
	order sets to integrate with cardiovascular clinical paths.			
1e.	Continuous care clinical paths for clinic management of chronic disease states			
	• Participate in the IHI initiative's to improve quality of care and decrease LOS, and expense for the surgical patient. • CHF pilot: practice guideline, order set • Partnership with clinics • Outcome indicators to be measured across the continuum of care.	1998–Ongoing		
1f.	Pilot new care management models			
	• Extended observation for heart failure • Work site risk reduction • Smoking cessation partnership.			
2)	Expanded service to referring and consulting physicians and clinics.	Ongoing 1998	1	Program Director, Service Line Personnel, Systems Manager, Outreach Coordinator, Cardiology, and CV Practices.

	• Expand, revise and improve Service Line activities to all Constituencies as needed:
	  • Scheduling • Pre-procedure routing
	  • Transfer service • Outreach services			

3)	Provide needed resources for each cardiovascular service:	Ongoing 1998	1	Medical Directors, Program Director, Administrations Department Directors, Nurse Managers, Staff, Steering Committees, Systems Managers, Cardiology and CV Practices.
a.	Analyze physical environment, patient and procedure volumes, practice patterns and department operations quarterly to determine cardiology program needs in all areas of service provided.			

Making Product Line Management Structure Work

The most important goal of the clinical product line structure is the collaborative relationships that must exist within the team in order to meet the organizational goals. For this reason, leadership is the key to success. I believe that effective leadership in this structure requires a partnership between the medical staff, senior administrators, and product line managers, standing together to lead the team toward goal attainment.

As Katzenbach and Smith (1993) told us in *The Wisdom of Teams*, a working group's performance is a function of what its members do as individuals, whereas a team's performance includes both individual results and "collective work products" that reflect the joint contributions of team members. Teams differ fundamentally from work groups because they require both individual and mutual accountability.

In a successful program, the commitment of team members is very evident. What are the key issues in developing high-performance teams? My physician partner and I use the techniques described by Katzenbach and Smith for all of our work teams. Since 1993 the CV work teams have become increasingly more autonomous and accountable for work assigned by the larger program team and self-directed assignments.

Choosing the right leaders for the program is the most important decision in organizing a product line structure. The leaders must be visionary individuals who can consistently lead diverse work groups toward a distant goal and gain commitment from varied stakeholders. The physician leader or medical director must be respected by his or her clinical peers and have credibility in dealing with all members of the medical staff.

The physician leader and the program operations director must be respected by team members and practice honest, open communication. These leaders must demonstrate collaboration in their daily relationships with each other, their peers, administration, and workers in the trenches. Product line leaders must also demonstrate commitment and integrity to the people they are expecting to lead.

Commitment begins at the top. A program that is supported by the organization's administrative leader is visible, accountable to articulated goals, allowed to be innovative, and given a high level of autonomy.

Traditional medical staff and management leaders are not always the best candidates for product line leadership. Product line leaders must demonstrate innovation and risk taking, along with solid management and leadership skills. While management skills can be taught to leaders, leadership skills cannot be taught to all managers.

Components of Product Line Structure

The components of a product line are varied and can be complex; they may require that the product line manager develop varied skills. Some of these skills must be learned on the job, because formal education has not totally prepared managers for the new challenges at hand. In a CV product line, for example, there are program components that require development and management. Specifically, the operational components encompass preventive care, invasive and noninvasive diagnostic care, interventional or procedural inpatient acute care, and rehabilitation and outpatient continuum of care modalities.

The most challenging components are those that are not directly managed by the product line manager. Examples include surgical and operating room (OR) components, emergency department components, anesthesia, marketing and home care. Accountability for these services is held collaboratively with other department directors.

As mentioned earlier, in the first forms of product line management all of these elements were included in the individual program silo, which was a very costly arrangement because of the duplication of task and service for all product lines (such as separate ORs, housekeeping services, and so on). As health care dollars became less available, these structures became prohibitively expensive, and institutions either modified their approach to be more collaborative or reorganized in a strictly functional system.

Linking Components Through Matrix Management

There are advantages to the collaborative management approach, but matrix management has its own set of challenges. Traditional management boundaries become blurred, and turf issues can ensue. However, advantages such as shared goals, multiple perspectives, and division of labor, which lead to better outcomes, make the effort worthwhile.

In our product line, matrix management of shared program initiatives is governed by the collaborative team approach, and multiple directors share accountabilities. Examples of shared projects include the Chest Pain Evaluation Unit, the Congestive Heart Failure Clinic, and the Adult Cardiac Surgery initiative to reduce costs and improve outcomes.

In each of these examples, the initiative developed by the CV program must be operationalized both in areas that are directly managed by the product line operations director and in areas that are managed by other directors. For the Adult Cardiac Surgery Initiative, for example, the scope of involvement included the OR, intensive care unit, telemetry step-down unit, cardiac rehab, physician practices, anesthesia, and others.

These initiatives required many hours of staff time in collecting and analyzing data, influencing peers, redesigning work process, and teaching and learning new systems. The major cultural changes required in work redesign initiatives cannot and will not happen without the total commitment of myriad directors and physicians working collaboratively to make the necessary staff time available, to provide leadership for complex system issues, and to enlist the support of the medical staff.

Collaborative Management Through TQM and CQI

Our CV product line has developed a unique and aggressive approach to integrated quality and process improvement by establishing an interdisciplinary CV work team. This is a collaborative practice model that provides the governance structure for the program. Membership includes physicians from all disciplines who care for CV patients, nursing personnel, related departmental personnel, finance, information systems, quality and case management, data services, and administration. The team is led by the program medical director and facilitated by the program operations director. All clinical and financial performance data related to cardiovascular DRGs are analyzed by the CV work team and its staff. We particularly rely on outcomes data from clinical paths and clinical practice guidelines, as well as available related information, such as readmission rates, costs per case, disposition of care, morbidity and mortality, appropriateness of care, service quality, average length of stay, and severity of illness. Program and physician-specific performance profiles are maintained and continually updated. Variance analysis data and related information are utilized to develop action plan formats, which become work plans using the PDSA cycle. Implementation strategies are developed by case type clinical action teams (such as congestive heart failure and acute myocardial infarction) appointed by the large CV work team. Changes in clinical practice and processes that result from implementation of these action plans are then reanalyzed in a continuous improvement cycle. The diagram in Figure 5.2 depicts this structure.

Physician-related data is utilized for peer review and clinical practice improvement. The meeting to discuss physician-specific and aggregate medical practice data is held quarterly and conducted with a peer review format. All data is plotted on control charts, which has proven to be very helpful.

The CV program team meets quarterly to determine quality improvement activities and to review the progress of all clinical action teams. We consider this the most important meeting for all

**Figure 5.2. Cardiac Centers: Mercy and
Unity Hospitals, Allina Health System.**

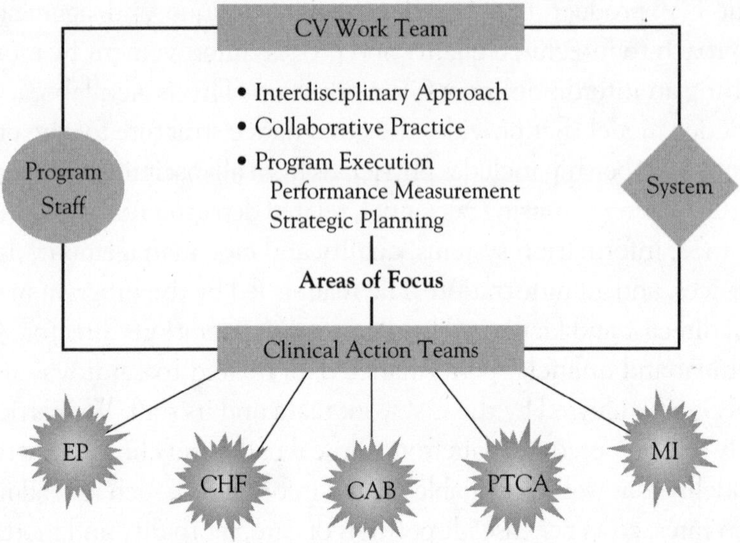

```
                         CV Work Team

                    • Interdisciplinary Approach
                    • Collaborative Practice
    Program         • Program Execution
    Staff              Performance Measurement        System
                       Strategic Planning
                              |
                        Areas of Focus
                              |
                     Clinical Action Teams

     EP                                              MI
              CHF        CAB       PTCA
```

caregivers and stakeholders, as this is how we monitor progress
toward most of our program goals. The team has a quarterly business meeting at which marketing and financial information is reviewed, and business planning is coordinated. We have a regular
monthly meeting schedule, with a consistent day and time for the
whole year, and rotate the peer review, quality improvement, and
business agendas.

The team's mission is to effectively and efficiently coordinate
the delivery of cardiovascular services to the communities we serve.
Again, mission and goals direct our efforts. To accomplish our mission of effectively and efficiently coordinating the delivery of CV
services to the communities we serve, we pursue the following goals:

1. To develop and implement "best practices" in care delivery to
   ensure quality outcomes

2. To develop and promote collaborative care models

3. To use a multidisciplinary, CQI approach for process improvement

4. To reduce variation in processes, systems, and practices

5. To foster innovative approaches to cardiovascular care

6. To provide responsible stewardship of resources

7. To collaborate with all Allina Health System delivery sites and providers to ensure integration of best practice methods

At the system level, the hospital leadership team represents the individual hospital on the systemwide CV steering committee. The vision and goals of the steering committee are reflected in each operating unit's business plans. Goals are articulated in these broad categories:

- Clinical care integration and clinical care model
- Resource stewardship
- Physician integration
- Marketing
- CV information systems

The vision and mission of the IDS is thus carried through each level of the organization.

Mechanisms to Achieve Program Goals

It is no longer enough for the product line to manage financial outcomes. In health care systems, managing patient outcomes within each setting and effective disease management across the continuum of settings and time (that is, clinical integration) is required.

When beginning to develop goals for a clinically integrated program, the first question should be, What is the most important "product" that we provide? Often, the laundry list of goals is overwhelming. Thus, the challenge and the value of this question is in focusing the team and helping it to set priorities.

Financial goals are the easiest ones; if we want to be providing the same services to our community next year, we need to meet our financial targets. In our market, we learned this lesson in the late 1980s. Despite the fact that we in Minnesota lead the country in cost containment, we still have a long way to go to be as efficient and effective as we could be.

In my consulting role, I travel to many hospitals around the United States. Based on what I have observed, I believe that we as health care providers have tremendous opportunities to improve the value we deliver to our consumers. Thus, my answers to the question about the most important "product" we provide is first, care management in our varied settings and, second, disease management across the continuum of care.

Care Management

Care management can mean different things to different professionals. Therefore, we employ various care management tools that the multidisciplinary team has developed over a seven- to eight-year time frame and that are now integrated into a solid care management approach. The tools include clinical paths and physician practice guidelines that have evolved over the years to become more comprehensive and integrated. We will soon achieve our ultimate goal of a computerized medical record that will automate the entire tool set.

The program team started developing clinical paths in 1989 as our first tools for care management. We moved from surgical case types to medical case types as our expertise grew. After a few years of analyzing variance from process and much experience with process improvement, the physician members of the team saw that the remaining visible variance was in physician practice. The first physician practice guidelines we produced was one for acute MI, quickly followed by guidelines for chest pain evaluation and congestive heart failure management. Preprinted order sets, quality indicators, and data collection tools for each set of practice guidelines completes the tool set.

The clinical paths have become CareMaps and are very different from the documents we first developed in 1989. We have learned to integrate many needed tools into the clinical pathway, including the problem list, expected outcomes at different points in the recovery process, the data collection tool for patient outcomes, the patient education tool for each case type, the preoperative checklist for each surgical case type or the preprocedural checklist for each procedure, the kardex information, the standard of care for each case type, and the physician orders for each day of the pathway. We also use the path format for preoperative testing and preparation and outpatient, rehab, home care, and clinic visits. Finally, we have developed self-directed paths for patients to use as a bridge from inpatient acute care to the outpatient setting.

Our paths have become sophisticated, comprehensive tools and are still the foundation of our care management philosophy. Moreover, these tools have become the cornerstone of CQI initiatives for the entire product line.

Case Management

Case management is another mechanism that we find key to the achievement of program goals, in the acute care setting and especially for disease management across the continuum. We employ clinical nurse specialists with master's degrees to case manage acute care patients who are "off path" (approximately 3 to 5 percent per case type). These case managers are consulted by the primary nurse when a patient needs more intense management.

As examples, cardiac rehab specialists case manage postcardiac event patients using a program that combines a path, outpatient visits, and individualized care plans to prevent readmissions and to establish solid self-care management skills. Smoking cessation clients are case managed by cardiac rehab professionals and respiratory care practitioners, both over the phone and in person. Our success rates for smoking cessation exceed the national benchmark.

Chronic disease state patients can benefit greatly from a registered nurse case manager to teach better coping mechanisms, self-care skills, exacerbation intervention, and reconditioning. In a three-month pilot with a congestive heart failure (CHF) clinic, we reduced the readmission rate for the pilot group by 100 percent and decreased the annual cost to the health plan by $325,000.

The pilot previously mentioned focuses on a partnership among a clinic with a large CHF population, a cardiology practice, the health plan, and the product line or program of the hospital. The "clinic" is held weekly at the large multispecialty clinic and is staffed by an internal medicine physician, a clinic nurse, and a cardiac rehab nurse from the hospital. Patients attend cardiac rehab at the hospital twice a week. During these sessions, they are assessed, taught, supported, and exercised by their RN case manager. The health plan has authorized payment for these visits for the pilot group.

Patients who are home-bound are visited by their home care case manager. Phone triage is handled by the clinic nurse involved in the pilot, as opposed to the regular triage system. Off-hours triage is covered by home care for these patients. The hospital has also arranged for free transportation for patients involved in the pilot.

We expect that strategies to help patients manage more independently with fewer acute care interventions will ultimately result in better patient outcomes at a lower cost for the most expensive chronic case types in the United States. As Bower discusses in Chapter Nine, our preliminary results suggest that RN case management is a powerful clinical integration mechanism and a key strategy for the future.

To truly achieve our goal of perfecting the disease management product that we provide to consumers, health care providers and health plans must better align incentives to promote resource stewardship and reward providers for appropriate utilization. Capitation, packaged pricing, built-in risk sharing, and strategies to share cost savings, although not yet common nationally, are essential to effective disease management.

Rapid Cycle Turnaround CQI

We have recently redefined the care of the adult CV surgical patient by combining two surgical groups' orders into one set and becoming much more aggressive in moving toward a four-day length of stay. We have participated, along with our system colleagues, in the Berwick's Institute for Health Care Improvement Breakthrough Series for Adult Cardiac Surgery. In October 1996, forty-one health care organizations representing over fifty cardiac surgery programs began working together to reduce costs and improve outcomes in adult cardiac surgery, as part of the IHI's Breakthrough Series (Berwick, 1996). Each organization participating in the collaborative formulated its own goals in ten selected areas:

1. Preoperative and operation room management
2. Anesthesia and perfusion management
3. Ventilator management
4. ICU resource utilization and length of stay
5. Patient and family education
6. Postdischarge follow-up and readmission rates
7. Catheterization to CABG time
8. Mortality
9. Database development
10. Atrial fibrillation prophylaxis and management

Through this collaborative, we have learned how to apply the technique of rapid cycle turnaround to our process and quality improvement work.

Rapid cycle turnaround is the latest strategy we are employing to improve care management. The technique uses all of the quality improvement tools we had already learned and applied, but it changed our thoughts about sample sizes and time-to-change cycles. The Plan, Do, Study, Act (PDSA) approach is applied at an accelerated rate, using small sample sizes. Our cycle times are two weeks in duration, rather than the three to six months we were accustomed to.

Applying this technique is a huge cultural change, and it requires a mature team whose members have a high level of trust in one another and are willing to take a risk on a new concept that may be contrary to their formal training. To organize this project, a six-member steering team attends three learning sessions three months apart, sets organizational goals (or "Aims," as the collaborative characterizes them), and mobilizes small work teams once they return to their own practice setting (Berwick, 1996).

Because of our solid program approach and product line organization, we were already prepared with our small clinical action teams to carry out this new approach. The small work teams were already high performing, motivated, and committed. Without additional resources we refocused some of the work and data collection in order to produce results every two weeks. This created high visibility to all team members, the administration, and the system as a whole. We have been participating in this project since October 1996, and our results to date have been extraordinary. Outcomes include a reduction in length of stay by more than two days, reduction in cost per case of approximately $2,000, improved communication and service to patients and families, and improved quality of care.

In summary, whether product line organization is viewed as a business, marketing, care or case management, or disease management strategy, there are three key elements to success: (1) employing a collaborative *team* approach, (2) using PDSA rapid cycle improvement techniques, and (3) making data-driven decisions. What differentiates a product line in a competitive marketplace is the ability to manage the experience of care for the consumer. In this scenario, the need for service excellence and high-level communication cannot be overestimated.

Advantages of Product Line Management

In a product line organizational structure, program goals flow more easily to tangible results and articulated outcomes. If one director has clear accountability for all the experiences of care of a group of patients, issues are much less likely to fall through the cracks. In contrast, a strictly functional organization often has boundaries that become barriers to providing needed optimal patient service.

Disease management strategies of the future require product line structures to effectively manage case types across the continuum of care. Areas that are typically not addressed by traditional functional management include (1) scheduling for smoother transitions of care from clinic to hospital, from hospital to hospital, and from physician to physician; and (2) preoperative or procedural contacts with patients to accomplish preregistration, assessment, testing, housing and transportation arrangements, education, social services, and spiritual counseling.

Accountability for the program's financial outcomes motivates the product line manager to develop strategies to improve costs per case that encompass several departments and services. The product line manager is given the incentive to "think outside of the box" and take more risks, as traditional ideas and methods often will not meet integrated goals for cost, quality, organizational, operations, and continuum of care initiatives. The product line manager is the only leader who receives the across-the-board cost per case reports and is accountable to improve these positions by engaging all of their partners to address their areas of individual responsibility. The product line model is an integrative structure that provides a more objective view of all of the essential components of any program.

From a work redesign perspective, product line management provides the opportunity to bring the management of several smaller areas under one director, which facilitates cross-training. Multiskilled workers can improve efficiency in related areas. Examples from our experience include training respiratory care practitioners (1) to perform EKGs on off shifts, thus eliminating the need for additional shifts of EKG techs performing only one function and (2) to remove arterial sheaths, providing a core group of experienced staff who are always available to remove sheaths, as opposed keeping a larger group of nurses competent. Finally, the centralizing of reception, scheduling, follow-up, and outreach activities for several related areas under one product line manager makes for both improved effectiveness and lower costs.

The clinical product line manager brings an essential perspective to marketing the service. In the absence of product line management, marketing is either ignored or left in the hands of the marketing department, with little input from the clinical experts. The best marketing concepts come from clinical experts with creative ideas to offer to their communities.

The incentive to bring more ideas to the table is probably the most compelling reason to consider product line management. Because of the overview accountability inherent in the model, high-level collaboration is required to meet the strategic goals, which taps the creativity of more stakeholders. As a result, the outcomes of this collaborative model are more likely to meet the goals of organizations seeking excellence.

Challenges and Disadvantages of Product Line Management

As mentioned earlier, the single most important ingredient for product line success is *leadership*, from both the medical and the administrative staff. Unfortunately, visionary medical staff leadership is the exception rather than the norm in many organizations. However, there are usually potential candidates who, if paired with the right operations director, can be developed into the progressive leader that product line organization requires.

When searching for the right individual to be a product line operations director, a host of qualifications must be considered that may not have been developed in traditional management positions. These qualifications include progressive management experience, strong team development skills, a record of fostering positive program development relationships with physicians, a strong strategic and marketing orientation, exemplary communications and presentation skills, the ability to thrive in a matrix management environment, creativity and risk-taking, and knowledge of health care economics in the specific market, including an understanding of its current level of evolution and what is likely to happen next. I also believe that a clinical background is an essential asset for this position, as I draw on my clinical knowledge and experience daily.

Product line leadership requires a high level of commitment and a passion for the product being delivered. Finding the right leaders is the greatest challenge and may sometimes seem impossible. Moreover, it takes many years to build a truly strong program, and some upwardly mobile managers may not be interested in staying in the same job that long.

Product line management is not well understood by all institutions and systems, as collaborative, matrix management is very different from traditional, functional department management. To change styles of structure, one has to be careful not to create new silos and to not add unnecessary cost with duplication of services. Many systems are not ready for matrix management and are uncomfortable with that level of ambiguity. It takes quite a while to become accustomed to the matrix model; communication must be very open, and a high level of trust must be established between all the players. Perhaps the most significant issue for traditional managers is the loss of control over the daily operations and services that are managed by other directors or by teams. It is difficult to accept overall accountability for outcomes when one can only influence the process, not manage it.

As Shortell (1985) has suggested, high-performance organizations are those that are committed to the extraordinary, maximize learning, take risks, create chemistry, have a bias for action, manage uncertainty, and create a strong culture. He also advised that we need to create strategies for high performance; ones that deliver high value care, innovation, growth, and a reputation for excellence. Experience has taught me that product line management can produce these results.

Conclusion

Product line management as a strategy for successful clinical integration relies heavily on flexibility and creativity. To create systems and processes for clinical integration the traditional organizational models must be abandoned. Product line management allows clinicians and administrators to come together to create more successful health care experiences for patients and families.

Product line management eliminates the boundaries that have created organizational barriers. The product line management teams share roles and collaborate at a level never before achieved. A high level of trust emerges, and all team energies are patient-focused; overall accountability is shared, resulting in improved outcomes and innovative models. The product line organization of the 1990s is the most practical, efficient, and effective way to address health needs across the continuum of care.

References

Berwick, D. (1996). Institute for Health Care Improvement Breakthrough Series for Adult Cardiac Surgery. Boston: Institute for Health Care Improvement Collaborative.

Katzenbach, J. R., & Smith, D. K. (1993). *The wisdom of teams*. Boston: Mc-Kinsey & Company.
Shortell, S. (1985). High-performing health care organizations: Guidelines for the pursuit of excellence. *Hospital and Health Services Administration*, July/August, 7–35.

Chapter Six

Strengthening Provider-System Integration

Robert B. Williams

The third type of integration essential to the success of organized delivery systems is individual provider-system integration. The drivers of the delivery system are the patients and the clinicians. By helping patients make decisions about their health, doctors greatly influence the selection of resources the system uses for the patient. Doctors are uniquely positioned to conserve system resources as well as to develop clinical programs that will sustain or increase clinical revenues. This chapter addresses key factors in achieving desired clinician collaboration for system success.

Clear Strategy, Vision, and Population Orientation

An organization that wants to form a partnership with physicians must have a clear picture of what it wants to be and how it plans to get there. There must be leadership and board commitment to involving physicians in the development and growth of the enterprise. The leadership, management, and providers must understand that the system is providing broad care to a population of people, not just acutely sick or injured individuals.

Understanding Physicians' Needs

Successful systems and their relationships with providers will be based on an understanding of the needs of patients, primary care physicians, specialty physicians, facilities, and ancillary providers, along with other stakeholders.

Traditional health care organizations and systems have been hospital-centric. While this observation may have become trite in administrative literature, it cannot be overstated.

Strategies for creating collaborative arrangements and financing mechanisms between physicians, other providers, and facilities rely on knowing what patients and their families need and want. Many hospital systems have ably assessed patient preferences for the inpatient setting and learned to more effectively meet the "customer's" needs and expectations. Systems that hope to engage physicians in system success must learn what physicians need and want. Learning about these needs and wants takes time and effort. As Covey (1989, p. 255) suggests, "Seek first to understand . . . then to be understood."

A key message to understanding the current physician mindset is that significant portions of the work of primary care physicians and sub-specialty physicians do not overlap. These two groups of physicians play essentially different roles in a system of health care. As systems mature, primary care and sub-specialty physicians are likely to understand each other's roles better. An important goal of a system should be to structure relationships such that these physicians understand and value each other's roles.

In most emerging systems, sub-specialty physicians do not fully understand the role of the primary care physician. This lack of understanding is a barrier to organizational development because hospitals have traditionally looked to the sub-specialty physician for leadership. Many physician hospital organizations (PHOs) are still suffering from this barrier. The desired goal is to help physicians see how they can help each other succeed. Understanding the needs of primary care physicians and sub-specialty physicians and finding ways to bring the two together will smooth the process.

Understanding Essential Ingredients of Success

One of the most important questions to systematically ask potential system physicians is, What do you think it will take for you to be successful in the practice of medicine? Asking this question of physicians will accomplish two tasks: (1) it will enhance trust with the physicians because it is unlikely that anyone has asked them this before, and (2) it will give the questioner important information about what your physicians need to partner with your system. In the context of this question, success is defined as the professionally gratifying delivery of quality health care and the achievement of financial goals.

In one collaborative independent practice association (IPA) established between academic and community primary care physicians, the academic center valued the opinions of the community physicians enough to assess these opinions. Many professionally developed, structured focus groups were conducted with primary care physicians of the same specialty. Not only were the IPA sponsors able to identify what these physicians perceived as factors critical to their success in the coming days of managed care, but they established the basis for future relationship building—prior relationships were fragmented due to several years of neglect of community physicians. In addition, we learned which configurations of hospital linkages would be valued by the primary care physicians in the market.

From our experience, physicians are likely to identify a combination of clinical and financial factors as essential to their success:

1. *Clinician is positioned to provide quality services.* Doctors want to be working in an environment in which it is easy for them to provide quality health care to their patients. Doctors and other health professionals are motivated by a desire to be more competent—to do a better job for their patients. The challenge for the system is to reinforce by word and deed that it shares that desire for competence. Simply assume that we're all in the same boat (administrators and clinicians) and want to be better at what we do.

2. *Sufficient resources are available.* Doctors want to know that they have sufficient resources to take care of patients in a timely manner. Will their office sites meet their expectations for safe, clean, inviting, and efficient workplaces? Will the office be designed for

easy patient access, comfortable waiting, personable staff, appropriately trained staff, ample size and number of exam rooms to facilitate appropriate patient volumes, and support staff cross-trained and willing to handle clinical and clerical tasks? Administrators must demonstrate to practitioners that they want to understand what it takes to create a satisfactory workplace. Physicians must demonstrate their desire to meet the administrator's need for efficiency.

3. *Access to quality and available sub-specialty and diagnostic services*. When their patients need diagnostic tests and further evaluation, can these services be accessed in a reasonable time and without heroic effort by the referring physician? In one multispecialty group, the neurology practice was notoriously slow in responding to requests for consultations. The neurologists had not caught on that their lack of availability represented a serious lack of service expected by physicians and patients. On some days, a call to the clinical office was routed to the voice mail system! Consequently, other specialty physicians in the group routinely referred patients to neurologists in other groups.

Clearly, outmigration of referrals is a serious financial loss to the overall group. Identifying outmigration referrals can be a key investigative approach to identifying significant system problems. Barriers to reasonable access to referral and diagnostic services must be removed. Over 90 percent of the time, diagnostic tests and referrals should be satisfactorily scheduled without need for additional referring physician involvement other than ordering the test or referral.

Likelihood of Achieving Financial Success

Primary care physicians want assurance that they will have a diversely insured population of patients who consider them as their primary doctor. In this context, "diversely insured population of patients" implies that the patients attending a given practice are insured by multiple third-party payers so that changes by one employer or loss of a contract with one payer will be buffered by the remaining group of patients covered by other insurance plans.

Many clinicians say that they grow uncomfortable when more than 15 percent of their patients could "vanish" overnight.

The key to financial success for primary care physicians will be their ability to maintain a balanced patient population without having to expend too many resources in attracting that population. By helping to minimize physician time spent on negotiating multiple contracts and streamlining the management of enrolled patients, the integrated system can add significant value for the primary care doctor.

Sub-specialty physicians want assurance that a diversely insured population of patients will choose to come to them or will be likely to be referred to them by other physicians. The same value can be added to the sub-specialty practice. The key here is helping the physicians to identify which services they can and should include in the negotiated relationships and to link their services with both primary care providers and individual patients seeking sub-specialty services.

Meeting Priority Needs First

Highly creative and intelligent managers and leadership physicians can brainstorm and make a list of many interesting needs and services that might be appealing to practicing physicians. However, successful systems will focus their efforts on the high-priority current needs first, while looking ahead to identify the priority future needs of their doctors.

System leaders often identify a unique service or feature that the system has developed for other users and apply this idea to what they perceive the doctors need. While many of these innovations are clever and may be "nice-to-have" services, partnering relationships with physicians are built on meeting high-priority needs for business success and quality patient care.

Many academic centers, teaching hospitals, and larger community hospitals place a high value on their continuing medical education programs. It is tempting to assume that this will be of significant value to potential system physician partners. While CME is of value to physicians, it is readily available to most practicing physicians. It does not qualify as a high-priority service in today's context of ensuring successful practice in our competitive environments. On the other hand, as markets develop, the transformation of traditional CME to continuing education that is linked to state-of-the-art comanagement of diseases and positions physicians in the system to provide more cost-effective, quality care might indeed be perceived as truly valuable.

Priority Physician Preferences

In our experience, in most developing markets, physicians' priorities can be categorized and ranked as follows:

1. An adequately insured patient population
2. Opportunity to share risk
3. Support for risk sharing (contract negotiation and contract management)
4. Incentives for performance (detail on compensation strategies without ownership; equity purchase performance)
5. Lifestyle enhancements
6. Pleasant and efficient physical plant

In more highly developed markets, in addition to the ongoing need for a population insured by multiple payers, the items further down the list emerge as higher priority.

Information systems are not on this list. While many physicians can understand and verbalize the need for information systems, until the delivery system is more integrated, the need for information technology is not perceived generally as a high priority. Such systematic enhancements will fall under the purview of the leadership group.

Opportunity to Share Risk

Increasingly, physicians recognize the desirability of assuming risk for a larger portion of the premium dollar. This recognition varies by physician characteristics such as age, type of practice (group or solo), current practice volume, and general level of risk tolerance. Physicians over the age of fifty-five tend to perceive less of a need to change the way that they do business. As well, physicians who are very busy in their current practice and have not personally experienced decreases in patient volume are less likely to appreciate the need to prepare for market changes.

Physicians who practice in groups are more likely to see value in assuming risk, possibly because in their group they have delegated a physician to oversee their contracting and have learned the value of investing focused effort into learning how to make the rules work for them. Also, their willingness to practice in a group represents their willingness to trade autonomy for the possibility of group efficiency.

Lastly, physicians are by nature risk averse. Why else would we choose to delay gratification for so long to complete medical school and residency? It is important to remember this personality characteristic when working with doctors.

Support of Risk Sharing

While more doctors recognize the value of assuming risk, fewer are comfortable in leading the process. This is where they find comfort in numbers and in working with people who have experience with risk and general business skills. The burden of personally negotiating contracts with multiple managed care companies has worn out many physicians, and they are left feeling like they have gotten the short end of the stick. How can you see patients all day long, review contract fine print, negotiate with the big boys, and have a chance of a favorable outcome?

Clearly, physicians see the value in negotiating from a position of strength. This strength is defined by a significantly larger group of physicians working together, coupled with professional contract negotiation experience. Any organizational structure that is well designed to provide these services can add value for physicians. The "professional" contract negotiator can even be a skilled physician who is dedicated to leading this process for the group. Early wins in gaining covered lives with favorable contract terms are key to building future cohesiveness for the system.

Subsequent to the acquisition of desirable contracts comes the immediate need for contract management. Anticipating this real need and having plans in place will demonstrate to the physicians the likelihood that the enterprise will continue to add value to the practice. The outcome of interest then becomes the number of covered lives. Not only is this number of interest to the physicians and their system partners; it is also of great interest in the marketplace. Managed care companies and competing networks will position themselves based on the perceived strength of your organization, largely based on your ability to deliver covered lives.

Incentives for Performance

As physicians come together and begin to share risk, they learn firsthand that their practice behavior will influence revenues. How can compensation distribution be designed to meet the goals of the organization?

As physicians have worked with multiple HMOs and been on the receiving end of payer-driven incentives, they have generally learned what they do not like. Incentives or performance-influenced compensation must be transparent to the physician. He or she must understand on a daily basis which behavior is being rewarded. The system will not succeed if it is too complex and therefore must be simple and straightforward.

For example, if a targeted outcome is an increase in appropriate screening mammography, the reward formula must not be so complex that the benefit beyond quality patient care is hidden to the clinician. How else can one desired outcome among many rise to the top of the busy agenda between doctor and patient?

Lifestyle Enhancements

Physicians value lifestyle-enhancing aspects of centralized groups. However, which ones they value will vary from locality to locality. Nightcall coverage, demand management, inpatient management for primary care patients, and other amenities may be the next steps that physicians want to take. One example of demand management is the use of nurse call-in lines to educate patients and encourage self-treatment, which reduces the number of patients choosing to visit the physician's office for simpler problems. However, such potential lifestyle enhancements must be assessed for the specific group. The clinicians have to see the value and be willing to "pay" for these services, as they will pay in one way or the other. Any service adds system costs that must be borne by someone.

Pleasant and Efficient Physical Plant

If the system takes over the management of the physical plants of the physicians' offices, physicians will want to make sure that their local office is attractive to their patients and that there are no system impediments to their individual productivity. Ample numbers of staff, examination rooms, and so on must be maintained. While such a statement is common sense, it must be recognized as a high-priority preference for almost all physicians.

Influencing Physician Behavior

There is a growing body of knowledge about interventions that can influence physician behavior. In my experience, physicians are predominantly motivated by a desire for greater competence. Most doctors and other health care professionals want to be better clinicians for their patients. Therefore, the most effective way to help physicians meet their need for continued improvement is to provide them with the tools to do their job better.

As with most human systems, myriad conditions and interventions influence physician behavior. Schwartz and Cohen (1990) identify knowledge and attitudes, regulations, peer pressure and feedback, incentives, and the overall environment as the strongest predictors of the diffusion of medical innovation.

What works in influencing physician behavior? Experience and literature suggest that the interventions that follow are among the most effective in changing physician behavior.

Meaningful Feedback

One of the most effective ways to influence physicians' behavior is to supply fair, comparative peer feedback. In the case of concerns about resource utilization, referral rates, length of stay, and performance of prevention and screening tests, this can be a helpful method for physicians to focus on behaviors that are worthy of increased effort (Greco and Eisenberg, 1993).

However, feedback reported must be clear and concise, and it must use both visual and written messages. If you can't get it on one page, reconsider providing the feedback at all. There must be face validity to the report; in other words, the clinician must find the report to be generally believable. Small numbers of physician-specific sample sizes are a common source of physician mistrust of such reports.

Guidelines

In my experience, physicians favorably perceive the use of guidelines. However, they are now facing inundation with multiple guidelines from payers, professional associations, and government groups. This only adds confusion and leads to a sense of being overwhelmed.

Locally adopted and maintained guidelines are more likely to affect physicians in their day-to-day practice. This does not imply that local physicians must develop the guidelines. Local endorsement of nationally derived guidelines is preferable. This provides an ideal opportunity for the emerging system to add value. Sponsorship of the physician guideline group and dissemination of the results will once again give the physicians tools for more effective practice.

More developed systems have sponsored disease management teams co-led by a subspecialist and a primary care physician and made up of other providers: nurses, nutritionists, health educators, and others. This configuration foretells the true potential of well-integrated systems: providers working together to provide quality care to a population of enrollees, delivering the appropriate amount of resources at the least costly site.

Education

Traditional, didactic medical education has proven to bring about little detectable change in physician behavior. This predominantly passive form of diffusion of innovation is easily forgotten in the barrage that hits doctors daily. Educational programs should be needs-based; make sure that this group of doctors perceives the need to learn about this topic.

Principles of adult learning theory and effective instructional design principles should be applied. Adults learn best under project-oriented circumstances. This is best accomplished in the didactic setting by establishing a personal anchor, through techniques such as identifying the last few cases in which they experienced the topic at hand. Provide focused materials designed to reinforce the objectives of the session.

System Support

The system can provide other tools to help the physician accomplish desired outcomes; generally, systematic solutions to recurring problems are better than repeated independent solutions. How can the integrating system manage diabetes most effectively? With physician endorsement, can we use computer reminders to reach goals of retinal exams, foot care education, and hemoglobin A1C measurement. Traditional medical education has not rewarded physician participation in population-oriented systemwide solutions to patient needs. Residency training programs generally reinforce a "buck-stops-here" approach to management. Doctors learn that if they don't do it, it might not get done. Integrating systems have a great opportunity to introduce systematic solutions to population- and disease-specific problems. How can our system help doctors ensure that almost all of our female patients ages fifty to seventy-five receive annual screening mammography? In the midst of a busy symptom-driven week, can we expect physicians to accomplish this intervention for every indicated patient?

Regulation

We can expect health care regulatory review to increase greatly over the next ten years. The system will be responsible for communicating regulations and ensuring that system members obey the law. Clear information and communication about risk will help to achieve the desired behavior.

Fear is a great motivator. Individual physicians will continue to be personally responsible for their clinical and billing behavior. Once again, I think the combination of motivation and helpful tools can lead to improved compliance.

Incentives

While physicians are highly motivated to be more competent, we are still human and do respond to incentives. This is entirely appropriate as long as the incentives are not likely to lead some of us astray.

Once clear performance goals have been established, key behaviors should be linked with financial or other incentives. The completion of preventive services can be rewarded. Base levels of clinical productivity and superior levels of productivity can be rewarded. Conventional wisdom suggests that 25 to 30 percent of compensation should be at risk to effectively influence a physician's practice behavior. Regardless of the level that is set, the behavior and reward must be transparently linked.

Using Financial Links to Strengthen Provider-System Integration

Tight financial linkages lead to tight organizational alignments and performance. While carefully structured financial relationships can assist in reaching system goals, this it not always the case. How these arrangements are implemented and how physicians are included in the governance and decision making process are equally important.

Clearly, all such financial relationships should be evaluated by legal counsel in the context of the local and regional market. It is still illegal to establish financial relationships with physicians that are designed to fill beds or ensure referrals to the parent institution. In the late 1990s, the trend is toward closer regulatory scrutiny of such relationships.

Successful system leaders are looking for ways to create the glue that helps physicians buy into the overall system goals. Physicians must feel that they are part of an organization or are partnering with an organization that is committed to meeting their needs, as described in the preceding sections.

Paying for Physician Administrative Time

As a general rule, the physician's time should be valued. What are the relative value units for time and effort spent in planning, developing, and learning how to practice more efficiently and effectively? While institutions cannot generally afford to pay the opportunity costs for the time that a physician could be spending in providing direct patient care, physicians must know that the system values their time. This translates into payment for significant work time on boards and committees that develop the principles by which system objectives are met.

In my experience, this equates to budgeting the equivalent of a locally respected honorarium for time of physician participation in such meetings. Consequently, quorums are usually met and physicians find it easier to give up that extra evening if they perceive their organization is placing a demonstrable value on the activity. For physician leadership, this means paying salaries for full time or part time physician positions.

Physician Employment

Employing physicians may be the best way to "control" them. However, if the system indeed desires to control physicians, it should go back to the drawing board and rethink the system's mission and values. Even employed physicians need to be seen as partners and collaborators.

Generally, physicians can be employed by purchasing their existing practice or by hiring the physician to work in existing system practices. However, there are innumerable accounts of systems and hospitals losing tens or hundreds of thousands of dollars monthly on newly acquired physician practices. In many markets, systems have not demonstrated the ability to manage newly purchased practices. Often there is a fundamental lack of understanding that the core business of a physician practice is different from the production model of an acute care hospital.

Furthermore, most of the acquisitions were structured simply to acquire the practice and failed to clarify the new rules for productivity and performance in physician practice. In almost all cases, the prior incentive for productivity was removed and the physician behavior changed. In traditional private practice, especially in the fee-for-service setting, where most U.S. physician practice patterns have been established, physicians have to meet monthly costs before contributing to their own salary. Consequently, each reimbursable service provided after meeting expenses contributes to their take home pay. Understandably, their incentive to come early, stay late, and be very available to see patients has been directly linked to their income. Why is anyone surprised that this incentive to come early, stay late, and be very available is significantly reduced after these acquisitions?

Similarly, with newly hired physicians, the same incentives are likely to come into play. With this relationship, it may be easier to establish new rules because it involves direct employment and is not tied to negotiation about the price and terms of acquisition. The message is to separate the new practice relationship from the actual old practice acquisition and be very explicit about expectations of employment. Get clinicians involved in establishing these new rules.

Physician Equity in Joint Ventures

Once again, regulatory concern about paying physicians for referrals has gained intensity. Hospitals that have offered physicians ownership in the hospital or system have come under scrutiny. While definitive action has not been taken, legal counsel should review any such arrangements with special attention to local and regional market issues.

Physician equity in joint ventures for management services or contract negotiations may avoid such close scrutiny and provide opportunity for creating system alignment. If physicians own part of the organization that manages certain aspects of their practice, especially managed care contract negotiations, they may be more likely to invest their time, effort, and practice behavior toward understanding how they and the system can succeed in providing care to populations of enrollees.

Exclusive Contracting Entities

Achieving some level of exclusivity in contracting is an objective of organizations created to negotiate and manage contracts. There are at least two boundaries to consider in establishing this exclusivity.

The first is the boundary between physician autonomy and potential gain from centralized services. Once again, we are faced with historical states rights-versus-federalist issues. Early in the process of coming together, physicians are wary of putting all their eggs in one basket. One approach is to agree on a period of time for which participating physicians will give exclusivity to the negotiating organization for contracting with a given managed care payer. During the time period, if the entity successfully negotiates the contract, then the participants are bound by the new agreement. If the time period expires without a negotiated contract, the participant physicians are free to contract with the payer independently or with other entities. In one primary care IPA, the time period for exclusivity was sixty days. This allowed ample time for negotiation but did deter the doctors from independent negotiation after the period.

The second boundary issue concerns antitrust issues and the legality of excessively long time periods. Likewise, the sixty-day time period met this requirement in the preceding example. Helping physicians establish contracting entities that allow for some degree of exclusivity is a first step for some systems to demonstrate to physicians the value in linking more closely with a given organization. The hope is that the entity will perform well, and the physicians will be willing to take the next steps to integration. This approach is valuable in a market that is not changing too rapidly because it gives the doctors time to incorporate change into their lives, rather than be forced to change overnight.

Other Financial Links

Another common method of financially linking with physicians is the creation of support entities to assist physicians in operating the practice, managing personnel, billing for services, contracting with managed care companies, and other services.

Purchase of Practice Management Services. Building management service organizations (MSOs) to make practice life easier for doctors is a strategy that can work; however, it again depends on leadership understanding the core business of physician practice. Additionally, physician equity in these types of organizations equates to their level of buy-in. If doctors own, participate in, and are well-served by these service organizations, they will have a stronger allegiance to the integrating system.

Nonexclusive Entities (PHOs, IPAs). Many observers see PHOs as providing little value to physicians. Sponsoring hospitals may gain value from presenting the perception of physician support while the local managed care marketplace matures. However, integrating systems need more than loosely affiliated physicians' involvement in the contracting process. Once again, exclusivity is a desired characteristic.

The conflicting needs of primary care physicians and subspecialty physicians in PHOs contribute to difficulties in getting much accomplished. Lacking strong market pressure, these physicians are unlikely to agree on how to share premium dollars.

System support for single specialty IPAs, multispecialty IPAs, or other contracting entities is one way of building experience and the potential for collaboration on primary care, sub-specialty, and facility contracting needs. During this phase, it is important to look for ways for the entities to work together for joint contracting experience (that is, what premium dollars can primary care physicians, sub-specialty physicians, and facilities gain for the provision of across-the-board care to people enrolled in a given health plan). Again, this approach works best when there is time for give and take in the market.

Hospital Staff Membership with Participation in Committee Structure and System Process. There are some physicians who will remain loyal to a given institution and its emerging integrated system regardless of contractual relationships. Although the number of such physicians is dwindling, do not underestimate the power of including the medical staff in the process of designing the new system. The desire for individual professional competence and the desire for a system that will serve the needs of the greater community are still strong priorities for many, many doctors.

Conclusion

Systems that succeed in integrating physicians will spend a lot more time in building trust and collaborating with physicians than they think is necessary at the outset. So much of what determines success is based on human relationships. With the right mix of heads around the table, you will have little trouble in figuring out a valid strategy. The hard work will be in the communication and implementation of the strategy. My advice is to get physicians with the right characteristics to join in leading the process. Then tell them the rules and give them the tools to achieve the common goal of greater competence in taking care of the people whose commonwealth you share.

References

Covey, S. R. (1989). *The 7 habits of highly effective people*. New York: Simon and Schuster.

Greco, P. J., & Eisenberg, J. M. (1993). Changing physicians' practices. *New England Journal of Medicine, 329*, 1271–1274.

Schwartz, J. S., & Cohen, S. J. (1990). Changing physician behavior. In J. Mayfield & M. L. Grady (Eds.), *Primary care research: An agenda for the 90s* (Conference proceedings). Washington, DC: U.S. Department of Health and Human Services, Agency for Health Care Policy and Research.

Part Three

Clinical Integration Practices

Chapter Seven

Achieving Information Systems Support for Clinical Integration

Teresa Mikenas Jacobsen and Maria Hill

A major component of clinical integration is the management of information as it relates to promoting health, treating illness, and managing disease. As integrated delivery systems (IDS) assume responsibility for covered lives, they must manage the wellness and illness information for both the population and for the individual.

Rapid, continuing development in the information systems arena has created opportunities for the IDS to deploy state-of-the-art technology. These systems are used in gathering, processing, reporting, and accessing information from all points of the continuum. Thus it is important to recognize the breadth and variety of information systems and technologies required to manage care.

Systems and technology used to support clinical integration is often found within the area known as clinical systems. *Clinical systems* is defined as "the field of management, systems/technology, and use of information as related to the delivery of care and the management of health. The common denominator throughout clinical information systems is the patient (a commonly used term regardless of the wellness or illness state of the individual)"(HIMSS, 1996, p. 2).

These systems and technologies have transformed the ability of a health care system to provide clinical information everywhere and every time it is needed and to everyone who is appropriately associated with the care and management of the patient or member. For many clinicians, this mind-set for clinical information (everywhere, every time, everyone) has become the unifying vision for information systems.

Understanding Clinical Integration Requirements

Care coordination is a highly sophisticated, interdependent process that plays a central role in clinical integration. It combines clinical, fiscal, and information science data to manage the continuum of health care to achieve best practice. For each population, *best practice* is defined as the achievement of optimal clinical outcomes at the best price, with the highest degree of patient satisfaction.

Three core components are integrated within the care coordination process: (1) clinical path and CareMap tools, with a concomitant variance management system designed to move to a documentation by exception philosophy and form a corporate standard of care by patient case type across the continuum; (2) case management, as well as other newly developed roles designed to promote clinical integration of care for complex patient populations over the continuum; and (3) collaborative group practices that assume accountability for outcomes of care for a defined group of patients over the health continuum.

Clinicians, as they articulate requirements to support the care coordination process, cluster their needs into three major areas: (1) a desire for an integrated medical and health record over the continuum; (2) ongoing support for the multidisciplinary plan and the record of care with clinical decision-making capabilities; and (3) the need to analyze and manage outcome data that support clinical practice changes for a population and information requested by outside reviewers.

Requirements for the Integrated Health Record

A very basic model of the integrated health record would contain longitudinal, critical patient or member information. This information, which helps clinicians manage care between and among entities within the health care enterprise, is paramount for clinical integration. This technology-enabled record ideally consists of key clinical and demographic data, which includes history and physical information; allergies; a list of problems; an inventory of clinical encounters, episodes, and referrals; test results; current plan of care; current medications; preventive efforts (such as pap smears and immunizations); and identification of the patient's primary and specialty physicians and case manager. This automated record is highly valued by clinicians.

This record of vital information is also valuable to patients. Patients and their families grow impatient with their caregivers when asked to repeat their history, allergies, problems, and medications with each encounter. This frustration is frequently articulated in terms of loss of confidence in and satisfaction with their care providers.

Although there are many different approaches, the integrated record is often made up of multiple systems and technologies, and the information does not completely reside within one system. The record consists of an advanced clinical system, the physical accumulation of specific clinical data in a repository, and a technology infrastructure, which connects additional systems and allows the retrieval of key information across the enterprise. The latter implies a logical approach toward data access in which the data resides at its source (that is, within the systems by which the information was originally processed), such as a physician practice management or a home health system that supports that entity's care process.

Requirements for Care Process and Clinical Decision Support

Ongoing care process support is the second area users need to manage and deliver care at any point of service. The requirements center around support for the care coordination process and clinical decision making. Care coordination process requirements focus on the ability to assess and diagnose the patient to facilitate accurate identification and utilization of clinical paths for that encounter, episode, or treatment period. These plans, in turn, integrate multi-disciplinary orders, expected outcomes, quality indicators, clinical rules (algorithms), and baseline and exception documentation. Information generated from these plans drive other applications and processes, including order management; cost, workload, and variance analyses; supply utilization data; and scheduling requests.

Likewise, clinical decision support is required to analyze information and create knowledge, often aimed at the individual patient. This may be articulated in various requirements that include the summarization of critical patient data (to support the management of exceptions to "normal" data); the integration of clinical rules with documentation, orders, and outcomes; the automation of alerts and reminders; and the capture of key outcome and variance data.

Requirements for Outcomes Management

Demonstrating effectiveness in coordinating care across populations through reporting outcomes is the third area of keen interest to clinicians, payers, and employers, as well to the IDS. Outcome information is "often difficult to define because it can relate to the following areas: organizational performance, clinical effectiveness, patient satisfaction, service quality, appropriateness of care, patient response to treatments, cost of services, efficiencies of services delivered" (Matthews, Carter, & Smith, 1996, p. 3).

Achieving automation can be very complex because of the varying types of data needed and the levels of effort required to gather, measure, manage, and monitor outcomes across a population. A broad array of information systems may be required to support outcomes management, as data may stem from the documentation process or administrative, financial, and claims databases. In some cases, there are niche systems that can support specific outcome types. For example, systems for specialty-oriented outcomes, such as cardiology and wellness-focus outcomes assessed with the SF–36, exist in the marketplace.

The Planning Framework

The challenge for the IDS is to define which systems and technologies are needed to support clinical integration within the enterprise. A useful approach to meet this need is the development of an information systems (IS) strategic plan, which has been successfully employed to examine IDS needs and acquire clinical systems. This framework provides a vital mechanism to identify IDS-wide priorities, allocate funding, and provide key resources in addressing the coordination of care as a continuum.

Initiation of IS strategic planning must be based on a clear understanding of the enterprise's strategic business plan, the IDS's future vision, and its strategic business and clinical drivers. Planners must have access to a clear-cut business plan that provides future direction; they must also understand clearly the factors that externally drive business decisions in order to create linkages with IS and articulate how information systems will support those business needs. Identification of these drivers should be based on an understanding of key customers (patients and families, physicians and clinicians, employers and payers), their needs, and the potential role that information systems play in meeting those needs.

The ability to produce a robust IS strategic plan also depends highly on clearly articulating clinically based information system goals, analyzing continuum-based reengineering efforts, and understanding care coordination mechanisms. Reengineering care coordination processes is a given if the IDS is to achieve clinical integration.

The planning effort must broadly define functional and technological requirements for clinical IS support, derived from these reengineering and care coordination activities. Requirements can then be translated into IS projects, budgeted, and prioritized for selection and implementation. Not surprisingly, clinical requirements often dictate several key system projects for the IDS.

Concurrently, effort must focus on understanding the legacy (current) information systems in place; specifically, the levels of user satisfaction, current funding of technology, and adequacy of the network communications infrastructure. This analysis provides the foundation for preparing strategies that recognize previous investments, the culture of the organization, past experiences with information system projects, and readiness to proceed with clinical systems and technologies.

Upon understanding the "where-we're-going" aspect (business direction) and the "where-we-are" aspect (current IDS and IS status), leaders within the IDS must develop their vision for clinical systems and its corollary strategies. A clear vision for clinical systems is required in order to gain key stakeholder commitment. Not all executives understand patient care and its management, so extra care is needed in creating the important linkages of why systems for the care process are needed to support strategic activities such as outcome reporting and demonstrating cost-effectiveness to prospective customers, as well as achieving a computer-based patient record.

In developing the clinical systems strategy, an understanding of the both the current IS environment and the operational readiness of clinical areas is essential, in relation to clinical systems vision. For example, realizing the vision of a computer-based patient record may require the leveraging of current ancillary systems (such as lab or radiology), procurement of advanced clinical systems and a clinical repository, the implementation of a network infrastructure, and standardization and linking of care delivery processes and data across the enterprise.

Next, the information systems organization evaluates the missing IS pieces of the clinical systems puzzle and predicts which system solutions are likely required to complete the vision. System decisions, derived from these requirements, must be linked to business and clinical strategies in order to establish priorities and sequence of procurement activities. Funding must be allocated and approved at the board and executive levels.

As these clinical systems are highly dependent on a solid technology infrastructure in order to achieve clinical integration across the IDS, clinical selections are often sequenced after an infrastructure foundation is set in place. In essence, technology becomes the "glue" of the enterprise and links core processes together. This is best illustrated in the following vignette.

Enjoying marketplace dominance, a pediatric health care organization focused on how to develop their own IDS for long-term survival. Among clinicians and executives, recognition was growing regarding the need for primary care approaches, which dictated strong, longitudinal care coordination strategies, for this niche population.

Physicians' and nurses' desire for a new integrated health record was growing, to help manage this population of patients quickly and effectively and to improve the ability to locate and access numerous previous care records during acute illness episodes.

Clinicians envisioned a highly developed computer-based patient record, and the organization's efforts aimed at process re-engineering were well underway. A strong legacy hospital information systems (HIS) and sophistication in care coordination was evident in advanced clinical systems throughout the critical care areas. Clinicians and executives decided to supplement the legacy systems with an advanced clinical system throughout the enterprise. Executive and stakeholder commitment and funding were prevalent.

The information systems (IS) department also initiated major networking infrastructure efforts to ensure intranet and Internet access to the integrated health record and pilot to support primary care and specialty care access via referrals. Multiple opportunities exist to leverage access to information to and from other information systems across the continuum.

System Selection and the Vendor Marketplace

The IDS evaluates the evolving vendor marketplace and their current and planned IS environment, and it defines the system needed to fit across many organizational entities. Often this definition of scope presents a major challenge, because decisions must be made about both the applications being sought within a clinical system selection and the IDS entities to be included in the implementation plan.

The Clinical Systems Marketplace

Myriad vendors claim to fit in the clinical systems field. Traditionally, entity-specific systems, such as HISs and ambulatory and home health system vendors, have often evolved to offer clinical systems functionality and care process support; however, there is broad variation in the depth and breadth of system functionality these vendors can provide across the enterprise. Even ancillary system vendors (such as lab, pharmacy, or radiology) have also seen major market opportunities to offer both clinical and ancillary support. They too stem from a long legacy of hospital and clinic support and vary widely in their availability to support the care delivery process across a broader continuum.

Since the late 1980s, advanced clinical systems have appeared in the market, often designed by clinicians to manage care robustly and to support clinical decision making. These products have rich functionality (as defined in the requirements section), and their vendors are aggressive in developing systems and applications to support multiple points across the care continua for which there is solid evidence of success. The advance clinical system vendors, in general, are most likely to support both the care coordination process and clinical decision support needs. Some of these vendors are also focused on creating a clinical data repository for collecting key clinical data about a patient or member over time.

The IDS Selection Process

Within the selection process, both care process support and clinical decision making are extremely important issues to clinicians. Although both are valued, physicians are most likely to prioritize clinical decision support capabilities at the expense of process support. On the other hand, case managers, nurses, therapists, and other multidisciplinary team members highly value planning, documentation, and outcomes support for their care process with the patient.

How does the enterprise find the right vendor "partner," whose vision is synergistic and who can offer the strongest, most complete clinical functionality across the continuum? Although the selection process can be fairly straightforward within a single organization, the practice variation and unique regulatory needs between and among entities within the health care enterprise can make finding the right system a daunting task.

The shift from a single focus (such as the hospital or the home health or physician's office) to the enterprise level has created additional complexity in system selection and implementation, because both the care process and decision support goals must be integrated across the care continuum. This complexity may be at its peak when standardization and integration of processes have not yet occurred; however, there can still be agreement regarding the scope of the systems applications and the clinical requirements.

Difficulties quickly arise during selection about how to handle overlap between entity-specific systems and clinical systems. Entity-specific systems, such as physician office or ambulatory clinic systems, are required because of the high degree of operational, administrative, and financial support needed within a particular organization. What muddies the water is that some clinical system solutions, specialized for those environments, may have different strengths than a preferred IDS solution. These "hybrid" products are often the result of mergers and acquisitions between two just-mentioned vendor types.

This approach can compromise the ability to integrate and coordinate care if systems integration is not carefully planned and managed. Multiple clinical systems, in different entities across the IDS, compromise the ability to standardize care delivery and information concerning the outcomes of that care.

Let's look at an example of the selection challenge. A group of hospitals came together quickly for survival. The newly merged enterprise was not well defined, and overall care coordination strategies were sketchy. The enterprises' executive team did not fully understand the overall business and clinical drivers in the marketplace. Several entities already had completely independent business plans and were implementing different approaches to coordinating care.

Operational consolidation was occurring quickly, and previous efforts in clinical automation had met with a variety of results. Politically, clinicians across the enterprise were requesting highly visible executive commitment and a common vision for clinical systems. Clinicians, from various areas within the hospital, were driving the need for the IS planning process. A much-needed IS plan was initiated to organize the diverse IS efforts that were diluting key resources (time, money, and people).

Management attention was given to the development of an achievable clinical systems vision and consistent goals for care coordination. Support from key corporate executives, which translated into commitment and funding, backed the vision and goals. The vision centered on capturing key clinical information across the continuum and on automating care coordination, to demonstrate population-based outcome management. The selection process, which was underway, was refocused to define clearly the scope of an advanced enterprisewide clinical system, and funding was reexamined to accommodate this change. A coordinated effort to prepare clinical operations for implementation was initiated.

This enterprise was attempting to automate both care and outcomes management across their continuum. As their focus was containing cost and coordinating care, their selection and implementation centered around inpatient settings, closely associated on-site clinics, and specialty areas (such as obstetrics) with integrated inpatient and outpatient services.

Physician offices needed access to clinical information but could not agree on what clinical support was needed within their practices. Regardless, the benefit of physician access to the inpatient and outpatient data was highly valued and perceived by the physicians as an overall win to the enterprise. Home care had already purchased and implemented a clinical support system; yet they badly needed access to inpatient data as patients were transferred to them at a growing rate.

As this example demonstrates, one or more entities are likely to be ahead of the others in their ability to successfully implement clinical systems for use in an IDS. They will often become champions throughout the IDS and align the IDS efforts for both the clinical IS support and the operational change required.

In the final analysis the ability to progress with selection and implementation of clinical systems will depend on the degree of operational readiness. The degree of challenge involved in implementing the new system will depend on several factors: (1) how ready the enterprise is for standardization of care coordination processes; (2) whether critical paths have been developed and applied; and (3) the extent to which those paths have been integrated with the documentation process. These readiness factors are major predictors of successful implementation.

Determining Operational Readiness
for Advanced Clinical Systems

Operational readiness is defined as the time an IDS is prepared to successfully support an automated solution for the care coordination system. This occurs when clinicians apply the basic principles of care coordination to all patients cared for within a defined scope of practice; that is, that every member of the health care team uses an integrated plan and record of care; documents by exception; tracks, analyzes, and uses variance and financial information to modify plans of care for an aggregate group of patients; and remains focused on outcomes (see Table 7.1).

Therefore, to accomplish care coordination for groups of patients and prepare for automation, the challenges include (1) standardization of multidisciplinary plans of patient care over the continuum by

Table 7.1. Operational Readiness: Self-Assessment.

Criteria	Institution/Agency	No	In Progress/Needs Improvement	Yes
A vision exists for clinical integration, care management, and clinical systems.				
All major constituencies have a basic understanding of care management.				
Executive management prioritizes care management program and IS resources for advanced clinical documentation.				
Infrastructure is established for care management to include definitions, format, policy, and guidelines and language.				
A program manager is present at each site.				
Strong interdepartmental cooperation exists between care management and IS.				
Integrated strategic business, care management, and IS make plans.				
Clinical pathways are implemented and monitored for several case types.				
Physicians lead and participate in path development, use, and evaluation.				

Table 7.1. **Operational Readiness: Self-Assessment.** (*continued*)

Criteria	Institution/Agency	No	In Progress/Needs Improvement	Yes
Collaborative teams are actively involved in using case mix, cost, quality, and variance information to change practice.				
Paths are developed as core of documentation system and integrated with charting by exception.				
Outcomes are identified, and a system is in place to track the financial, clinical, functional, and satisfaction data.				
Variance processes and systems are in place to record, collate, report, analyze, address, and re-evaluate data and care practice issues.				
Dedicated, flexible, and knowledgeable IS staff members solve technology issues.				

case type, (2) development of consistent documentation and variance management systems, (3) conceptual development of clinical decision support for both individuals and groups of patients and (4) identification and management of outcomes across the system.

Development of Infrastructure

Due to a combination of factors, including the differing requirements and initiatives of each entity within the IDS, the varying needs of patient groups, the unique focus of each clinical discipline, and data demands from internal and external groups, automation of care coordination and the documentation system is both extremely important and complex. Establishment of an IDS executive-level steering committee is an excellent strategy to meet these demands. The committee's charge is to bring leaders and managers within the health system together to create a vision and infrastructure for care coordination across the delivery system.

When merging organizations into an integrated delivery system the issues faced at first appear overwhelming. The central steering committee is charged with examining the major elements of a path system within each institution, the success of implementation within each institution, and the similarities and differences between the institutions with the ultimate goal being creation of a central organizing system.

The work performed by this group includes obtaining executive commitment to employ clinical integration through care coordination strategies. The commitment includes (1) creating and implementing corporate clinical paths, (2) developing a variance management system that integrates with the CQI structure, (3) empowering collaborative group practices through provision of collated data and services to assist with analysis of data, to make efficient and effective programmatic changes in patient care,(4) dedicating resources to reengineer the documentation system as the core process for data collection and reporting, and (5) developing a strategic work plan to automate the integrated health record.

Uniformity in Standards, Format, Definitions, and Implementation

The committee must outline the standards for the care coordination system and define all pertinent terms for tools that may be used in the integrated system, including but not limited to practice guidelines, clinical algorithms (a decision tree format depicting the presentation of key symptoms and values with actions to be taken), and clinical paths and CareMaps (see Chapter One for definitions of these terms). Each tool can be used, and critical values can be integrated into the paths (Kleinman, 1995). The focus for this chapter is clinical paths and CareMaps.

Although many acute care facilities have embraced development and implementation of clinical paths, these efforts frequently have not included standardization of tool format and language across case types. Before moving to automation, members of the committee must evaluate the uniformity in path format across the system, the consistency in clinical language used within the paths, the variance indicators selected and monitored, the degree of success in using the path system to manage patient care, and the system for data management. The next step is to create the corporate framework developing the vision for the IDS.

A sample policy is created to provide guidelines for development, implementation, and evaluation of paths. The policy outlines the multidisciplinary and multiagency members to be included in development, the literature to be reviewed to demonstrate evidence-based practice, the objectives to be realized with implementation, and the standard indicators to be tracked. As an example of a standard indicator, the committee might decide that a discharge or transition plan will be established for every patient within four hours of admission to an acute, subacute, or home care setting.

A standard format is also created that includes the problem statements, the elements of care categories (assessment, consultations, treatments, and so on), and the outcome statements. The group is challenged with developing a format that standardizes care, yet flexibly allows for both regulatory requirements in traditional care settings and specialty clinical population needs.

Defining acceptable terminology to be used for interventions and outcomes creates consistency of language among providers. Language can be a tough issue to resolve. How will each discipline's language be integrated (medicine, nursing, physical therapy)? Indecisiveness and conflict will impede the development of a data dictionary to enhance data entry, collection, and management across both provider disciplines and patient case types within the health system. The steering committee must decide to support both standardization and the reliability and validity of data collected.

Clinical Path and CareMap: Core of the Medical Record

The committee must decide whether the tools will be a permanent part of the medical record and the core of the documentation system. If the membership determines that the path is the central organizing device, reengineering of the record must ensue. This group then determines the relationship of the path to the medication administration record, the breadth of multidisciplinary charting, and the depth of normative standards by discipline in order to convert to a documentation by exception philosophy (Hill, Broad, & Rampetsreiter, 1995). Attention must then turn to integration of the variance management system. Questions the committee will grapple with include how to create a simplified record and decrease the amount of information each discipline records while accommodating those disciplines' unique identity and accountability, and how to ensure access to the tools and record outcomes of care.

Establishing Corporate Level Outcomes

Outcomes are the criteria selected to measure performance of the integrated health system. Categories of outcomes are traditionally identified by external stakeholders such as patients, employers, payers, community interest groups, regulators, accreditation bodies (such as NCQA, HEDIS, JCAHO, MDS, or OASIS-B), and internal stakeholders (physicians, nurses, and executives, and so on).

Performance measures are traditionally divided into the following six categories: (1) external customer satisfaction; (2) functional outcomes; (3) clinical process and outcomes; (4) financial performance; and (5) marketing and strategic business advantage, and (6) provider satisfaction. The foci in the path process are functional, clinical process and outcome indicators. Examples of system outcomes that may be incorporated into the clinical path system include absence of symptoms of nosocomial infection, absence of injury due to a fall, ability to return a demonstration on medication administration, and patient-perceived pain control.

The committee will assist in identifying the indicators to be used for internal and external benchmarking, the mechanisms for deploying selected standard outcomes to paths, and the variance analysis process. It will also outline the procedure for the addition of outcomes by patient population over the health system. For example, certain case type–specific indicators may be required throughout the system. For heart failure, the appropriate use of ACE inhibitors is generally tracked in all health settings.

Variance Management Systems and Using Data to Change Practice

The steering committee must also create the vision for the variance management system. Simply defined, variance is the difference between what is recorded on the path versus what is actually happening as care is delivered to the patient. While every exception should be documented in the record, the key questions for the committee are, What should be tracked and continuously monitored? Which indicators reflect efficient and effective care delivery?

The committee must make decisions regarding the variance management processes, which are outlined in a policy statement. They must also create standard report formats and distribution

mechanisms and design the integration with quality and performance improvement processes.

At the same time, the committee will be intuitively designing
variance entry, collation, reporting, data display (integrated data
relationships), and requirements for software to support the variance management system. A successful variance system will provide the following: (1) variance information from all patient points
of contact; (2) user-friendly data to providers; (3) accurate data
from integrated databases; and (4) assistance to clinicians in instituting practice changes that benefit the patient and family and
health system in cost and quality.

Assessing Integrated System Readiness: A Case Study

Three financially successful not-for-profit community hospitals, a
large home care agency spanning several counties, and several
physician office practices had merged to form an integrated health
system. The health system had formed an acute care–based intera-
gency committee to investigate computerization of the documentation system. The committee had developed a document outlining
desired features for clinical automation solutions in patient care delivery, as the precursor to a request for information. This step was
taken to organize the project over the health system. The next step
was to hire two consultants to assist the committee in evaluating
their readiness to select and implement an automated solution to
documentation of patient care.

Obstacles to Program Success

Independent efforts to develop paths had occurred at two of the
three hospitals prior to the merger. One institution had developed
an automated practice guideline application. The guidelines were
case type–specific and were used to guide patient care. Driven by
the inadequacy of the care planning and order entry function of the
current software application, a second hospital had established a

budget and committee to select an automated documentation solution. These independent efforts were arrested by the merger. Key players involved in these independent efforts served as participants on the system-level committee; however, home health, ambulatory care, and the subacute settings were not represented. Committee members remained committed to their institutional and discipline-based needs and had difficulty transitioning to an integrated delivery system perspective. The committee struggled due to lack of a dedicated leader at the executive level, a strategic work plan, and an understanding of the link between documentation and development of a data management system. As time passed, several influential committee members became frustrated by the previous time and effort invested in creating agency-specific requirements documents and in evaluating vendor software. Moreover, despite their selection recommendations, executive level sponsorship remained unclear.

A commitment to clinical path development and implementation existed in all agencies within the integrated system. However, the agencies differed in the number of clinical pathways developed and the level of success in implementing the pathway system. Multidisciplinary development of the tools occurred in each agency, but use of the tools as a document for the patient record varied. In all settings the physicians interpreted the paths as guidelines rather than permanent records of care delivered to patients. Simplification of charting in the medical record, both within and across agencies, was in its infancy. Additionally, variance tracking existed in one organization, but the information gathered was unreliable and therefore not used to change practice. All facilities lacked a well-developed infrastructure for the system (an active steering committee, a dedicated project manager, and an established collaborative group practices meeting regularly to discuss the paths, variances, and results of indicators tracked).

Different models for case management existed in each agency. The role and function of the case manager varied from utilization management, discharge planner and case expediter, to clinical case manager coordinating care over two settings. Due to the varied job expectations within the integrated system, the case managers had difficulty articulating and agreeing on automation needs to support their practice.

Case Study Recommendations and Lessons

The consultants recommended the following actions:

- Realign institutional priorities and demonstrate executive level commitment, leadership, and resources for the clinical path and clinical information system development.
- Expand the steering committee membership to include the postacute continuum and ambulatory settings.
- Develop a strategic work plan for the development and integration of care coordination and information technology across the enterprise.
- Establish a corporate standard for path development; standard language sets for problems, interventions, indicators and outcomes; and a consistent process for variance management.
- Establish physician leadership in path development, implementation, ongoing evaluation, integration into documentation, and selection of automated advanced clinical and documentation system.
- Create and use paths across the health care continuum.
- Select and develop demonstration sites to implement the advanced clinical and documentation applications using the principals of care coordination.
- Integrate variance management, data management, and the quality and process improvement systems over the episode through establishing collaborative group practices. Act on the variance data to change practice.

- Develop ongoing communication and systemwide goal development, education, and marketing efforts at all levels in the health system.

The advanced clinical and documentation system serves as the data management tool for clinical efficiency and effectiveness. The documentation process thus becomes an extremely important vehicle for clinical and financial performance review and ongoing continuous quality improvement at individual patient and aggregate levels. Therefore, evaluation of the documentation process and use of information software as an enabler of care delivery over the continuum is critical to achieving clinical integration.

Conclusion

Achieving information systems support for clinical integration is possible within the integrated delivery system environment. It requires a clear understanding of strategic business direction, care coordination goals, and the interrelationship of key initiatives such as reengineering, IS strategic planning, and advanced clinical system projects.

Patient care executives and providers must create the vision and support required to achieve a sound process for longitudinally coordinating and evaluating care of the patient and the population across the enterprise. This process directs activities toward developing uniformity of paths and outcomes, standardizing the medical record to integrate paths, and designing a variance management system to provide information about practice.

The chief information officer, with IDS executives and key clinical stakeholders, formulates an IS plan rooted in strategic business and clinical direction. Understanding the IDS's future direction, as well as its current clinical environment and culture, executives can create a meaningful clinical systems vision and strategies that support clinical practice across the different entities. Clinical IS strategies span multiple systems and technologies, both existing and leading-edge. The scope of new systems must clearly articulate functional requirements and related applications, as well as the entities impacted by the selection. Rapid changes in health care and in the systems marketplace often require vendor partnerships that will help the IDS formulate its best clinical solutions, given its clinical vision, current IS environment, and entity-specific needs.

Operational readiness assessment becomes the key step that links the enterprises' ability to integrate the newly acquired systems to a highly functioning process of care coordination. Operational readiness becomes a key determinant in success, as the redesign of processes for planning and documenting care must take place before implementation can proceed. Not surprisingly, system implementation is greatly slowed or halted if the enterprise and its entities are not ready. The marriage of care coordination and IS activities is vital to the success of clinical integration initiatives.

References

Healthcare Information Management Systems Society (HIMSS). (1996). *Guide to effective health care clinical systems*. Chicago: Author.

Hill, M., Broad, J. & Rampetsreiter, C. (1995). Integrating critical pathways and documentation by exception. In L. Burke & J. Murphy (E's.), *Applications in charting by exception* (pp. 175–178). Albany, NY: Delmar.

Kleinman, J. (1995). The physicians new agenda. In K. Zander (Ed.), *Managing outcomes through collaborative care*. Chicago: American Hospital Association.

Matthews, P., Carter, N., & Smith, K. (1996). Using data to measure outcomes. *Healthcare Information Management, 10*(1), 3–16.

Chapter Eight

Clinical Paths and CareMaps

A System-Level Care Management Strategy

Susan Robertson

Achieving clinical integration of patient care, the coordination of primary care, and specialty services within a system culture is the challenge facing all integrated delivery systems (IDS) today. The challenge becomes even more daunting as new partnerships are developed overnight, mixing academic and community, private and public, unionized and nonunionized staffs and cultures (Scott, 1997). Many IDS are experiencing rough transitions as they struggle to integrate staff, normalize labor relations, and create a common "system" culture.

Several key clinical integrating mechanisms have been identified to facilitate this transition at a regional system level (Conrad, 1993; Gillies, Shortell, Anderson, Mitchell, & Morgan, 1993). One of these mechanisms, care coordination, involves the creation of system-level protocols for different clinical conditions (such as pneumonia, stroke, hip replacement). When implemented effectively, the protocols lead to clinically integrated practice patterns. These protocols, or clinical paths, have been used successfully since the early 1980s as a tool for horizontal integration, to coordinate a patient's care within one hospital episode. Creation of clinically integrated practice patterns throughout a regional health system, however, requires clinical protocols for managing the care

I would like to acknowledge the contributions and support of J.S.T. Gallagher and the senior administration, quality management, and case management staff of the North Shore Health System.

of particular health conditions across a widening continuum of set-tings and services (such as acute, subacute, home care, and reha-bilitation) (Conrad, 1993).

This chapter outlines steps to successful development, imple-mentation, and evaluation of clinical paths and CareMaps through-out an IDS. Network-level strategies and support structures are described that foster both vertical and horizontal integration of care processes. Action steps are outlined as recommended approaches based on my experiences as an internal consultant in a large IDS and as an external consultant on care and case management to var-ious organizations, systems, and service lines.

The Road to Clinical Integration

As the administrative director of Quality Management in the North Shore Health System (NSHS), my job was to facilitate the implementation of clinical paths and CareMaps across all system sites, in conjunction with ensuring that regulatory compliance, pol-icy and procedure standardization, and performance improvement processes were in place in each facility. After a successful pilot and 100 percent implementation of CareMap methodology at the sys-tem's flagship, North Shore University Hospital, CareMaps were identified as an effective patient resource management strategy that would decrease the variability of care for case types within a multi-hospital system and provide coordinated, cost-effective care to patients across the system. In 1995, CareMaps were prioritized as a system-level care coordination strategy, and the pilot staff and the process were integrated into the corporate- or system-level Quality Management Program and Department. The approaches used in the initial hospital were drawn from experiences reported by oth-ers in the literature.[1]

Lessons learned from our pilot project and initial CareMapping experiences have been incorporated into the strategic plan of what is now the NSHS. These lessons are inherent in the action steps outlined in this chapter for CareMap implementation across an integrated delivery system. A brief overview of the size and structure of NSHS is included to set the stage and rationale for the action steps that follow.

North Shore Health System

Between 1994 and 1996, North Shore University Hospital grew from two hospitals (a 705-bed teaching hospital and a 240-bed community) to ten hospitals (over 3,400 beds), which are geographically dispersed throughout Long Island and Staten Island. These institutions are tightly linked to the system through ownership or sponsorship and help to support the NSHS's strategy to become "the integrated health care provider of choice" in this region of New York. Presently, the NSHS is one of the largest IDS in the Northeast, with a market area that includes the 7.5 million residents of New York's Nassau, Suffolk, Queens, Kings, and Richmond counties.

The ten inpatient facilities include two university teaching centers and eight community hospitals. In addition to the ten hospitals, two long-term care facilities, four home care and related service providers, four rehabilitation centers, and numerous ambulatory care sites and controlled physician practices comprise the NSHS. The scope of services provided across these sites is quite extensive and encompasses all clinical specialties, with the exception of transplants and burn treatment.

Five of the hospitals are owned outright. The remaining hospitals are linked to the system through a sponsorship agreement that allows them to keep their boards for an agreed on number of years; however, the NSHS is the sole voting member of those boards and can fill vacancies or add members as necessary. This sole voting capacity is essential for systemwide managed care contracting.

One of the greatest facilitative factors in developing this extensive hospital network has been NSHS's commitment to enhancing the community in which each hospital is located. As opposed to many networks, in which smaller community hospitals are often closed or used to "feed" the flagship hospital, the NSHS provides system services across the entire community that enable each hospital to continue to serve the community as before and offer new services based on community need. For example, two of the community hospitals are located less than five miles from each other. All obstetrical services and complex medical-surgical patients were moved to one hospital. The second site has become a state-of-the-art short-stay surgery center with ophthalmology, laser, and orthopedic specialties and a new pain management program. These changes provide the community with a broad range of new services, in addition to combined traditional programs.

Successful Implementation at the Site Level

In any change process the initial phase involves letting people know that change is imminent. Communication diminishes fear of the unknown and allows individuals to begin to accept proposed change. As each hospital or facility joins our system, they begin to learn of the benefits, from clinical to financial, they may realize as a member. The benefits include twenty-four–hour neonatology coverage, systemwide ambulance service, savings from group purchasing and insurance, and system-managed care contracting. CareMaps are also marketed as an effective method of decreasing length of stay, enhancing team communication and patient satisfaction, reducing resource use, and improving documentation and JCAHO compliance. With this introduction, the stage is set to present this concept to the local leadership.

Obtain Top Administrative and Medical Support

While an IDS can establish network or corporate strategies and policies, it is the local administrative and medical leadership who initiate and sustain change within their organizations. Therefore, any new process or system to be implemented must have support from these top leaders that is tangible and evident to staff. The administrator must decide when the facility is ready to begin the major initiative of implementing CareMaps.

Each site administrator generally has a working knowledge of who the motivated, energetic, internal leaders are and can be helpful in assigning these key personnel to the CareMap initiative. Additionally, this individual site administrator can set the stage by providing education and information to the department directors to engage their support and enthusiasm for the process. In today's competitive market, busy managers must be convinced of the worthiness and expected outcomes of a new process before they will undertake one more function. Administration must therefore clearly define the purpose of developing CareMap tools for the organization and set expectations for staff involvement, use, and evaluation. They may choose to sit on the steering committee if one is established, or they may receive progress reports during department head or performance improvement meetings. The most important facet is their verbal, unwavering support.

Similarly, medical leadership also has to be willing to actively support this initiative. The Medical Director must be committed to the initiative and willing to address medical staff concerns about CareMaps.

Active Physician Participation Key

No discussion of clinical pathways or CareMaps would be complete without discussion of physician response toward this process. As each new hospital is approached to implement this methodology in the NSHS, some members of the medical staff will voice resistance. The term *cookbook medicine* is derisively applied as physicians express their feelings of loss of autonomy and control.

Several processes have been implemented to encourage meaningful physician participation in CareMap development and usage. First, education is provided to new house staff during their first weeks of residency, and they are encouraged to actively participate in CareMap creation (that is, to prepare the literature review as a learning experience). Second, information on CareMaps as the patient plan of care is now provided as part of the credentialing process. Third, as each CareMap is developed, it is signed by the directors of all services who will be providing patient care for the diagnosis it represents. When the map is signed by the director of Nursing, director of Physical Therapy, and director of Neurology, for example, in the case of a CareMap for stroke, this facilitates approval by the medical board.

A disclaimer statement is printed on each CareMap that describes the map as a general guideline that does not govern the provider's obligation to patients. It also states that the plan is revised and care is individualized as necessary to meet patients' needs.

The medical leadership (director, chair of the medical board, chiefs of services, division directors) need to be sensitive to the concerns of their peers and may even have concerns of their own regarding the use of these tools in their practice. Our Risk Management office devoted an issue of their quarterly newsletter to the topic of CareMaps, citing positive references of usage in malpractice cases. This was helpful for physicians at the flagship hospital; they felt that their liability concerns had been taken seriously and investigated by the legal department. Another successful strategy to diminish physician fears is to bring legal counsel to a medical board meeting. I asked a trial attorney to come to such a meeting at one of our community hospitals. He explained his firm's position on the benefits of having a CareMap in the medical record: especially for lay people, the CareMap presents a comprehensive picture of the team's plan of care. He reviewed local and national trends and spoke positively of the CareMaps developed by this institution. After answering a minimum of questions, the board voted unanimously to make the CareMap a permanent part of the medical record, thus enhancing its use and integrity by all clinical staff.

Medical support might be the most difficult to obtain, but it is the most critical. The administrator and medical leaders should spend as much time and energy as needed to engage the high-volume voluntary staff in CareMap development and variance analysis.

Educate Staff

Functioning as an internal consultant, I begin staff education with an overview of CareMaps and variance analysis sharing several examples of success from the pilot project. Staff from multiple disciplines are educated on the impact of CareMap use (for example, reductions in average and median length of stay, variations around median LOS, total direct costs of care, total units of service consumed, and ancillary service use).

Data on key quality indicators is shared to demonstrate that the impact just described positively affects quality outcomes (such as nosocomial infection rate, patient falls, decubitus rate, medication errors, returns to the ED in seven days, and readmissions within thirty days). It is important to bring in all managers (department directors), clinical and nonclinical, at this point to allow them to feel part of the process from initiation and to enhance ownership. The presence of the site administrator, or his or her introduction of the topic, is crucial to informing the staff of the significance of the topic and how it will help the individual site and influence their connection to the system as a whole. Staff inservices need to be provided around the clock and on weekends to capture part-time staff. Every clinical department and all levels of staff must be included. Secretarial education is crucial to compliance with retrieval and submission of variance records. Many hospitals educate every employee with the mind-set that health care consumers should be familiar with this methodology.

Each department director should be challenged to think of ways to incorporate CareMaps into their present processes and documentation. If the CareMap is to be used properly by all disciplines, it should replace all other documentation forms to prevent redundancy and lost or overlooked information. Most systems that have successfully implemented CareMaps as multidisciplinary care plans streamline the documentation process for their staff with the CareMap as the care plan and evaluation tool, with each discipline's progress notes detailing their patient assessments and interactions.

Within each hospital, every department (such as physical therapy, social work, respiratory therapy, or nutritional services) is encouraged to develop an internal manual to help their staff in using the CareMaps. The first step is to describe their scope of services or the types of therapies or treatments they provide to patients. Next, the various tasks or interventions performed in providing the particular therapy are delineated. Finally, outcome statements are generated for each therapy.

The greatest challenge to staff in all specialties is the move to outcome-focused reporting and documentation. Developing standardized outcomes statements for common therapies and interventions decreases frustration and teaches staff to think in outcome language. Eventually, staff become comfortable with this process and begin to develop more creative individualized outcomes. An example from physical therapy follows: therapy-splint fabrication (which would be entered under the treatment category of the CareMap), with an accompanying outcome statement, "Patient demonstrates correct use of assistive device and adaptive equipment." The physical therapist would date and initial this outcome when the patient achieves it.

Develop Experts

North Shore University Hospital utilized a unique educational methodology to implement our pilot project. As project manager, I joined efforts with four clinical service managers (RNs) who were hired to educate staff, develop multidisciplinary clinical paths (CareMaps), and analyze variance data from these paths for patterns and trends. All five nurses, who were prepared with either bachelor's or master's degrees, had clinical expertise in their particular service (medicine, surgery, ICUs/ED, maternal child health, or psychiatry). Each used principles of change management to assist staff in comprehending the concepts of case management and accepting the first wave of change in health care reform. The clinical service manager acted as a bridge between disciplines, fostering nonthreatening collaborative relationships (Eckett, Vassallo, & Flett, 1996). They functioned primarily as educators and consultants to hospital staff, working in collaboration with and facilitating multidisciplinary teams. Through staff inservices and daily rounds, the service managers role modeled care management behaviors and provided case consultation. Head nurses on each unit played a major role in this model, with the responsibility and accountability of working with the service manager to implement and support this process on their individual units. They continue to be the backbone of any successful system. Acting as care managers for their patients each shift, staff nurses assume a proactive, outcome-focused approach, enhancing their autonomy and accountability. In addition, as nursing staff collected variance data, they actualized performance improvement where it mattered most— at the bedside.

As the pilot project ended, the service managers were deployed throughout the first four hospitals who joined the NSHS to function as project managers and implement this process in the hospitals to which they were assigned. As the system expanded, a different approach became necessary. I and a new nurse hired in 1996 began to develop in-house experts at each of our new facilities. These staff are identified by the site administrator and are usually nurses from Staff Development or from Care Coordination or Quality Management departments. They are trained in CareMap development and implementation and make site visits to similar hospitals to see a system fully implemented. Channels of communication are opened and enhanced across the NSHS as staff seek information from more experienced sites in problem solving and best practices.

This approach is successful because site-specific staff feel more comfortable working with their known personnel on a day-to-day basis. Information is accepted from the corporate office, but feelings of autonomy are fostered through working with internal staff.

Provide Meaningful Information

To begin the CareMap process in each hospital, staff need meaningful data to provide direction for where to begin. Our System Quality Management Department supports this process by querying each hospital's databases to produce utilization management reports. A yearly report is produced that lists the top DRGs (diagnosis related groups) that account for at least 50 percent of the annual census. This report is used for prioritization in CareMap development.

A second report details DRGs with length of stay in excess of HCFA (Health Care Finance Administration) standards, which are set and used for Medicare patients. This information is used to trigger focused reviews on these diagnoses to identify major variance sources. As length of stay improves in each hospital, with successful CareMap implementation for high-volume case types, the second report on excess days becomes increasingly important and identifies areas for case management (see Chapter Nine).

Create CareMaps

Like many systems, North Shore uses the Center for Case Management model of CareMap creation (Zander, 1995). Multidisciplinary groups meet to discuss optimal care patterns for various diagnoses and, using a spreadsheet format, map out tasks and interventions on a day-to-day time line in the following nine categories of care: consults, tests, treatments, medications, diet, activity, team process, teaching, and discharge planning. This experience of multidisciplinary creation greatly enhances the efficiency of care by (1) triggering referrals and orders for tests in a timely manner, (2) focusing the team on the progression of patient care throughout the acute episode in terms of diet, activity, and medications, (3) breaking down patient education into manageable daily segments that are easier to comprehend and learn, and (4) ensuring that discharge planning begins on the day of admission.

It is also an excellent learning process that fosters respect for each discipline's unique knowledge and expertise and helps the team understand how truly interdependent they are in helping the patient achieve optimal outcomes. This same methodology is used at all hospitals, and creation meetings begin with a summary of the most recent literature review and professional society and government agency guidelines, as well as a review of existing practice patterns gleaned through chart review. It is best to have the findings of this review presented by a physician expert, who can give an overview of current best practices. In this manner, all professionals who are busy in clinical practice become updated on the latest advances in treatment for the diagnosis under discussion. The standard of care is elevated with an expanded knowledge base. One important rule has been established at each site: a CareMap can be created only when physicians attend and participate; meetings are canceled and rescheduled when physician attendance cannot be ensured. Some hospitals invite prior patients to these development meetings to share their experiences and offer suggestions for improvement. Patient input is invaluable to the busy team and can greatly enhance the entire process.

CareMaps are developed for the top ten volume DRGs in the first year of implementation. One key to success is to have staff see and use as many of these new forms as possible to shorten the learning curve and enhance their integration into the day-to-day process of each unit or site.

Establish Outcome Accountability. CareMap creation sessions can be facilitated in various ways. One technique is to have the team brainstorm the optimal immediate, intermediate, and discharge outcomes for a particular case type. The group would then map out the tasks or interventions that lead to these outcomes. Conversely, the group could develop the day-to-day time line and then overlay the outcomes after visualizing the plan of care. In either case, it is imperative to establish during this phase which discipline is going to accept responsibility for assessing and evaluating each outcome. For example, in a hospital with an active respiratory therapy department, therapists may volunteer to assess a patient's readiness and ability to move from a handheld nebulized aerosol treatment (which requires staff administration and mixing of medications) to a handheld metered dose inhaler that is self-administered in preparation for discharge.

When a discipline accepts responsibility for an outcome assessment and evaluation, they commit to perform this function for all applicable patients so a systemic process is implemented. Nursing staff should not sign off on this outcome then, but any team member or care provider should call the respiratory therapist if documentation of this skill is not addressed in a timely manner. The director of Respiratory Therapy should likewise monitor staff performance and compliance.

Identify Key Clinical Markers for VAR Documentation. As the team creates the most efficient time line for patient, family, and staff behaviors to occur, another strategy that can be of great benefit at this stage is to identify key clinical markers. Markers may be either process- or outcome-based and consist of transition points or critical events within a CareMap that the team determines to be vital to successful completion of the episode of care. These are the areas from which variance is captured. (This methodology will be described in detail under the system-level implementation section.)

Educate Patients

During the CareMap creation phase, a patient-friendly version of the CareMap is created for many case types. These easy-to-read educational tools map out for the patient and family, in lay language, daily interventions they should expect from the health care team. They also contain suggestions for patients to contribute to their own care and recovery, for example, by drinking a certain amount of fluids after a particular test or operation or increasing ambulation daily. In our experience, sharing this plan of care with patients greatly helps to decrease anxiety and encourages and motivates patients and their families to participate actively in their treatment plan.

As the multidisciplinary team examines its process and improves upon it, they may decide to create an entire package of educational materials in conjunction with the CareMap and patient version. Our Pediatric Asthma Path team developed seven separate one-page discharge instruction sheets for each type of possible discharge therapy for asthmatic children—from peak flow meter use to chest physical therapy. Having instructional forms to refer to helped parents feel more comfortable and capable of taking care of their child at home. In addition, these tools helped to facilitate a safe, effective discharge in a shortened length of stay.

CareMap Implementation

Implementation of CareMaps achieves two goals: (1) care planning tools are standardized for all patients across the institution; and (2) CareMap documentation that combines tasks and interventions with desired outcomes provides a basis for outcomes-based practice. Successful implementation requires that the use of CareMaps becomes ingrained in the day-to-day operations of the unit. One major proponent is the use of the CareMap at the change of shift report reviewing patient progress and focusing the oncoming shift on outcomes to strive for. To achieve this goal, the nursing kardex has been removed (however painfully) in several hospitals, which leaves the CareMap as the primary tool or source of information. As long as the kardex remains, it inevitably competes with the CareMap, and staff do not discuss patient outcomes, only tasks. Several brave units undertook a pilot of the kardex-free process and finally convinced others to follow. Eventually, nursing managers and staff realized how much information was documented on a tool that is discarded upon discharge. The medical record is more complete when the CareMap is used alone, because there is less fragmentation of documentation. This assumes that the CareMap is a permanent part of the medical record. This is a vital step in the successful implementation of this methodology. Staff are too busy to complete documentation on any tools outside the medical record. Additionally, any process that is not incorporated in the medical record will not be seen as a worthwhile or serious initiative.

Lessons Learned

As each case type is being analyzed for care mapping, the team reviews and enhances the entire process of care delivery. One example of this includes the establishment of presurgical education classes for total joint replacement patients, during which patients meet with nursing, social work, physical therapy, and discharge planning staff about one week prior to admission. They receive instruction based on the patient version of the CareMaps and are screened for potential discharge needs. This is one of North Shore's first forays beyond the acute setting into the continuum of care.

This example also demonstrated that physicians become increasingly supportive of the CareMap process as they see new programs and services being developed for their patients as a result. The team's evaluation of common clinical scenarios or patient experiences helps in the development of CareMaps that capture the true progression of the patient throughout their stay. Another example involves the high-volume admitting diagnosis of chest pain, rule out myocardial infarction. This two-day path was expanded to include three possible conclusions: (1) the patient's cardiac enzymes are negative, and the patient is discharged for outpatient follow-up; (2) the patient's enzymes are negative, but they branch to a secondary path for continuing angina that might result in a cardiac catheterization or electrophysiology studies; or (3) enzymes are positive, and the patient branches to a myocardial infarction path for the duration of treatment.

A third example involves a prenatal CareMap that follows the mother for her nine-month antepartum period in the ambulatory clinic. This map, written in trimesters, reflects a complete history of the patient and her pregnancy and is delivered to the Delivery Room staff when the mother is admitted in labor to provide continuity of care and information. Once the mother has delivered, the vaginal delivery or C-section CareMap is added to the prenatal, so that the ambulatory and inpatient data are joined. Utilization of this CareMap set provides an excellent example of care coordination across an episode resulting in clinical integration of ambulatory and acute care. Similarly, inpatient CareMaps are being revised to reflect new transitions to alternative levels of care or services. For example, our Rehabilitation Planning Group is revising the CVA (stroke) CareMap to reflect a transfer to their inpatient program on Day Four following admission for patients who meet set criteria. New CareMaps are in development to reflect the plans and outcomes for this second rehabilitative phase of care, and they will continually expand to capture the entire recuperative process.

General CareMaps

In order to utilize the CareMap methodology and team mind-set for all patients, general CareMaps are developed by service (such as medicine, surgery, ICU, pediatrics, and psychiatry) that map out a generic admission process in each of these specialties. The overall HCFA standard for this service is used as the length-of-stay target. The CareMap content is developed throughout the patient's stay by combining the physician's orders with the multidisciplinary team's plans and anticipated outcomes for that particular patient. This results in an individualized plan of care for the complex patient admitted with several active diagnoses, for whom a case type–specific map would be inadequate.

Maintaining Site Individuality

As the NSHS has expanded, it has been important that the culture of each site be respected and preserved. Therefore, System Quality Management staff meet with multidisciplinary teams at each hospital and train their internal experts to develop site-specific CareMaps that reflect the local language and practice patterns (lab test abbreviations, diet names, and so on). Each CareMap has a well-substantiated literature review to validate its content. In 1996, NSHS hospitals moved to a new process whereby each individual CareMap, rather than just the first one developed at each hospital, is presented to the medical board for "ratification," to heighten members' awareness that CareMaps are used throughout their site, not just in their specialty.

Successful Implementation at the Network Level

Several factors contribute to success at the network level.

Establish a Unifying Mission

If a health care delivery system is to become truly integrated, an initial step is to establish a unifying mission and vision for the system that acts as a guiding principle in its development and daily operations. A clear and concise mission statement helps keep staff members focused on the job at hand with a vision for where the network sees itself in the future.

At North Shore, each of our facilities shares the system mission to provide the highest quality of care to patients; provide education to patients, families, staff members, and the community; participate in research to enhance medical knowledge and patient outcome; provide community outreach and services that improve the health of the communities we serve; and remain financially viable in our changing health care environment. With this mission established, CareMaps are readily seen as an effective network strategy in the pursuit of our vision to be the health care system of choice in our region.

The use of CareMaps allows an integrated delivery system to establish a single high standard of care that is effective and resource appropriate. In our competitive market, this is the key to survival: to be the provider of choice, providing high-quality, efficient care.

Provide Resources

For a CareMap system to be truly functional, it must be viewed as more than just the nursing care plan. Top leadership must drive this process. One motivating force behind acceptance of maps was our president, J.S.T. Gallagher, whose mandate and support of this effective strategy was crucial to its implementation.

As the use of CareMaps helped lower length of stay and resource use during our pilot program, Mr. Gallagher and the vice president of Quality Management realized that CareMaps also helped to clinically manage patients between the two focus points of admission and discharge. CareMaps also facilitate the multidisciplinary team interaction, flow of communication, and care planning mandated by the JCAHO (Joint Commission on Accreditation of Healthcare Organizations) standards and provided a social order for teams on the nursing units. In 1995, JCAHO added a new function for improving organizational performance that involves "Doing the right thing and doing it well." A second new function involves the continuum of care or the coordination of patient care across units, services, sites, or programs. CareMap methodology is a perfect response to the intent of these new standards.

This process was validated when the NSHS maintained all of the pilot positions and moved this staff to system-level positions. An additional nurse was hired as the system expanded, and technical staff have been added to support our centralized variance analysis efforts. This support and the provision of resources to each member site codifies the process.

Best Practices

On a system level, CareMaps are reviewed by diagnosis (such as simple pneumonia) and matched on two critical factors: length of stay and key clinical markers. The JCAHO and Department of Health have very clear expectations for the provision of the same level of care for all patients in a hospital, regardless of unit assignment or ability to pay. In using CareMaps as a systemwide methodology, we recognized that they are a helpful tool to develop a single standard of high-quality care. Matching the CareMaps on length of stay and key clinical markers helps to achieve this goal, because all sites performing joint replacement surgery have a CareMap with the same length of stay (based on the HCFA standards) and highlight key clinical outcomes or processes on the same day. Consequently, all patients who have a total hip replacement would be assisted out of bed on Day Two, unless a major variance has been documented.

For most of the community hospitals, services must be enhanced, (for example, physical therapy must be available seven days a week) to meet this standard of care. Improved services help to decrease length of stay and enhance the quality of care. Conversely, if the institution cannot provide this level of service, strategic planning would develop programs at the institution that are more appropriate to its resources. As each facility reengineers, they use the CareMap as an important methodology for mapping out more efficient processes, while maintaining optimal patient outcomes.

Patient Care Rounds

Another helpful process that is implemented in all system hospitals is multidisciplinary patient care rounds. These rounds are held two or three times per week on each patient unit and are attended by physicians, nurses, social workers, home care providers, and others in ancillary departments as appropriate to the population on that particular unit. These rounds are an excellent educational experience for house staff and students.

During rounds, three basic questions are asked regarding each patient:

1. Why is the patient here?
2. What are we doing for the patient today?

3. When is discharge anticipated, and have all the appropriate referrals and arrangements been made?

The team then discusses the answers and develops individualized treatment plans on the CareMaps.

When rounds are first implemented, it is difficult to get complete answers from the group. In many hospitals, patients are admitted with the infamous "rule out" menu (rule out myocardial infarction or congestive heart failure), or they are admitted with symptoms such as fever or dehydration, so the reason for admission is not clear for several days. In developing a more efficient process, it is important to work with the Emergency Department staff to obtain an appropriate admitting diagnosis. Additionally, it is helpful to have the medical and nursing staffs confer on the admitting diagnosis to ensure that the patient is on the proper CareMap, with the appropriate plan of care in progress within the first twenty-four hours of admission.

By discussing the second question, the team looks at its practice patterns and internal efficiency and ensures that all tests have been ordered and are being performed as necessary. This can also lead to discussion of variances as the care plan is modified to meet individual patient needs or adjusted to anticipated outcomes or target dates.

The third question is critical in establishing a safe and appropriate discharge plan for each patient. As each unit manager or service line begins to feel pressured about reducing costs and length of stay, it is easy to lose focus. It has been our experience that once the team knows why the patient is in and no longer can say what is being done on a daily basis, they move toward saying that the patient must be ready for discharge. The State of New York requires twenty-four hour discharge notification of patients, and this is a helpful regulation. The staff must be educated that a "surprise" discharge is not acceptable; rather, the goal is a well-planned discharge, with the patient's participation and agreement.

To monitor the effects of patient care rounds and subsequent LOS decreases, the NSHS carefully evaluates readmissions within thirty days of discharge and returns to the Emergency Department within seventy-two hours across all of its hospitals. Each readmit or return is reviewed to assess the appropriateness of the initial discharge plan. Any problems are referred to the appropriate department for peer review.

Establish Reporting Mechanisms

A space is provided for staff to indicate if the patient was discharged with no variances identified during the hospital stay.

Clerical staff in all NSHS hospitals remove VAR forms from patients' medical records at discharge and send them to the Quality Management Department at North Shore University Hospital–Manhasset on an ongoing basis. Forms are batched and electronically scanned by a data entry clerk. A statistician, using the raw scanned data, generates monthly and quarterly reports of variance on several levels.

The first level is institutionwide and provides a summary of discharges and average length of stay for all patients by month or quarter divided into four categories: (1) patients with variances noted; (2) patients without variances; (3) patients on single CareMaps; and (4) patients on multiple CareMaps. This report gives the site administrator an overall picture of patient flow during that time period. For example, if the hospital and its practitioners are functioning efficiently, 70 to 80 percent of patients are discharged without variance. For the 20 to 30 percent of patients for whom variances are documented, the majority of variances are physiological.

As each hospital implements CareMaps, it is interesting to note how variance sources change over time. Initially (that is, for the first six months), variances are split evenly between patients and families, institution and practitioners. As data are reviewed by the service line teams over several months to a year, and practitioner sources are fixed via education and feedback, the database begins to reflect patient physiology almost exclusively. This engenders performance improvement initiatives to improve outcomes for all patients or to identify high-risk patients. Subsequent levels of the variance reports provide more in-depth data on the variances that patients did experience.

The second level of analysis is by service line; all data from the units that treat patients from that service are aggregated and reported. This report details the percent of variance from each source type, with further drill-down for each source. If the cardiac service line finds that the majority of variances are physiological and from the cardiac system, a more detailed report may show that abnormal lab values or EKG changes were the problems identified within that subset. Reports presenting institutional, caregiver, and patient and family variances, with their sublevel categories (such as M.D. decision or patient refusing treatment), are also generated.

The third level of analysis is by nursing unit. Each unit receives the same kind of information as in the service line level, but aggregated by the individual unit. In this manner, managers and staff can see how their unit contributes to variance in their service line. Presently, we are looking at incorporating this variance data into each unit's report card of service, quality, and cost indicators. On this level, an additional report is generated that graphs the actions the staff takes to help patients achieve their outcomes. This report is prepared as positive reinforcement, to recognize staff's efforts and document their proactive approach. Head nurses are encouraged to display these graphs in the staff lounge.

The fourth analysis level is at the individual CareMap, and the same standard reports can be produced by diagnosis. This is a helpful level of reporting as new CareMaps are developed, allowing the team to examine the effectiveness of the new protocol and providing feedback to the team during the process of moving toward 100 percent implementation.

As CareMaps are implemented in each new hospital in the NSHS, the CareMap level and nursing unit level reports are generated monthly and quarterly. Data are shared with the team, and revisions are made to the CareMaps as necessary. As each site reengineers and develops service lines with CareMaps for all patients (such as cardiac, oncology, HIV), service level reports are produced monthly and quarterly, along with the housewide report.

As this methodology has spread across the system, a fifth level of analysis or reporting has become possible: measuring variance from the same diagnosis (such as C-section, chronic obstructive pulmonary disease) across the ten hospitals. This capability allows the system to do internal benchmarking and to identify best practices or, conversely, problem areas throughout the system. Through analysis of key clinical markers, data collection is standardized and focused on patient outcomes.

Performance Improvement

In 1994, North Shore University Hospital–Manhasset formed a performance improvement coordinating group (PICG). This structure is replicated at each system hospital and serves as an excellent mechanism for CareMap and variance integration.

A system-level PICG was formed in 1995 and consists of the chairperson of each site's PICG, the nurse executive, and the director of Quality Management, as well as NSHS staff from Quality Management, Risk Management, Infection Control, Pharmacy and Therapeutics, and Emergency Department Services. Chaired by the medical director of Quality Management, the system PICG is a multidisciplinary forum to provide each hospital's PICG with assistance and information to help coordinate and improve quality-related activities.

The system PICG provides a forum for analyzing and improving the care rendered by each institution. Information is shared among the institutions regarding best practices, quality outcomes, indicators, occurrences, and negative outcomes. All available quality-related data and information is aggregated and reviewed in this forum. One of the main goals of this committee is to promote the development of multidisciplinary standards of care via the CareMap methodology. Another is to receive, evaluate, and coordinate reports of performance improvement team activities and share out-comes and performance-related information. On both the site and system level, this has become the vehicle for reporting on CareMap development and variance analysis findings and corrective actions. The system PICG also reports to the Joint Conference Professional Affairs Committee of the board of trustees.

Support Structures

Networks or IDS are rapidly developing new system structures to meet the challenges of a managed care environment.

Managed Care. The Managed Care division utilizes CareMaps during contract negotiation to demonstrate the hospital's expertise in utilization management and specific efficiencies achieved. As we negotiate systemwide contracts, North Shore seeks delegation of utilization management responsibility from the payer, because of our experience and success in this area. Shared risk contracts are beginning to enter the New York market, and this greatly helps to integrate CareMap practice patterns and align hospital and physi-cian incentives more closely.

PHO/MSO. The NSHS maintains extensive relations with independent physicians and hospitals within the market area. These include over four thousand physicians on the medical staffs of the ten hospitals, more than 80 percent of whom elected to join physician-hospital contracting entities with the system. A system physician hospital organization (PHO) has been developed and is supported by local organizations at each hospital. The PHO and MSO (medical services organization) are two halves of the same entity. The PHO has been formed as an entity for managed care contracting, and the MSO manages the contracts. The MSO has contracted with the system Quality Management Department to continue to provide oversight and guidance for the utilization management function in each hospital. It is anticipated that as precertification is requested for provision of services, the CareMap would be faxed to the provider with the authorization.

Information Management. Information Systems (IS) represent another key clinical integrating mechanism at the regional system level. North Shore is moving toward a standard hospital IS throughout the network; by the year 2000, all hospitals will be linked by the same system. To join all sites, both inpatient and ambulatory, a clinical data repository will be established that provides a record of each care episode and tracks utilization and outcomes over the continuum. This repository, together with a master patient index, will provide a life-to-death record and ensure the tracking of patients across system services.

A computerized patient record is planned for the future. Through electronic access, CareMaps will be actualized at their highest level, enabling clinicians to customize expediently each patient plan of care.

It is anticipated that information exchange mechanisms can also promote clinical integration. One such mechanism, Physician Profiling, is in place across the system to provide individualized practitioner feedback regarding costs, clinical outcomes, and patient satisfaction. This information is educational and allows the physician to examine his or her practice against that of local peers and national benchmarks; it is not used for credentialing purposes. The data highlight variances in practice patterns and resource use and can encourage compliance with CareMap guidelines. Severity-adjusted software is being purchased to allow for more accurate comparison.

Another information exchange mechanism in place across the system is the Distance Learning Network. This equipment provides for teleconferencing and is utilized for grand rounds and educational seminars. Numerous clinical education programs are reflected in systemwide initiatives or meetings, many of which are broadcast to multiple sites over the Distance Learning Network. Several specific clinical processes have been targeted (such as pressure injury prevention and treatment, or fall prevention in all care settings), along with organ systems (nephrology case conferences) and patient management (ICU Grand Rounds, CareMaps). As discussed in Chapter Ten, this is another excellent mechanism for the development of system-level practice patterns (Conrad, 1993).

Centralized Laboratory. One of the greatest opportunities for integration through IS may lie in our newly centralized laboratory. This state-of-the-art center will provide services for eight hospitals by 1998, using total laboratory automation robotics. Through its IS, the centralized laboratory will standardize all instruments, reagents, policies, procedures, training, performance improvement indicators, reports, and so on. Laboratory is a service that patients use in every care setting, and this system will standardize registration information and order set definition and reporting of results. Standardization mechanisms such as this replace the need for "local language." Again, CareMaps continue to be more tightly woven into the fabric of the organization and system as these types of standardization occur.

Conclusion

This chapter presented steps for the implementation of Clinical Paths and CareMaps across an IDS. Strategies to enhance success were presented for both the individual site and network levels. While struggling to integrate, systems must respect the individuality of their components as they strive for efficiency.

Lessons learned from North Shore Health System's experiences are shared to assist others interested in this approach. The keys to success lie in administrative and medical support. Clinical staff enjoy multidisciplinary team interactions and appreciate more efficient and effective documentation tools. Patients are more satisfied when included in their plan of care. External forces in health care, (such as managed care, capitation, and risk sharing) demand that care coordination strategies such as CareMaps be implemented and used effectively. As the settings and services of care change and new continua are developed, IDS must continually establish new patient care processes. CareMaps are valuable tools that support multidisciplinary teams as they develop, monitor, document, and evaluate this care.

Note

1. I recommend two chapters in particular to readers interested in getting case management started in their facility, both from Zander (1995). Kyzer's chapter provides an overview of CareMap project management that describes the various phases in a CareMap implementation process (such as assessment, planning, design, pilot, implementation, evaluation, and integration). I experienced each of these phases as project manager from 1991 to 1993 at North Shore University Hospital, a 705-bed tertiary care teaching facility on Long Island, New York. Andolina's chapter is a step-by-step explanation of CareMap development and implementation. This process is based on the experiences of pioneers Karen Zander and Kathy Bower, who developed this methodology in the early 1980s at New England Medical Center in Boston.

References

Conrad, D. A. (1993). Coordinating patient care services in regional health systems: The challenge of clinical integration. *Hospital and Health Services Administration*, 38(4), 491–508.

Eckett, K., Vassallo, L. M., & Flett, M. (1996). A service manager model: Instituting case management. *Nursing Management*, 27(2), 52–53.

Gillies, R. R., Shortell, S. M., Anderson, D. A., Mitchell, J. B., & Morgan, K. L.

(1993). Conceptualizing and measuring integration: Findings from the Health Systems Integration Study. *Hospital and Health Services Administration*, 38(4), 467–489.

Scott, L. (1997). Can marriage of academic, community hospitals work? *Modern Healthcare*, March, 26–32.

Zander, K. (1995). *Managing outcomes through collaborative care*. Chicago: American Hospital Publishing.

Chapter Nine

Clinically Integrated Delivery Systems and Case Management

Kathleen A. Bower

Case management is an ideal strategy to make clinical integration real. This is particularly critical for individuals with chronic disease who are using an increasing portion of health care dollars. They are especially susceptible to issues related to fragmented care, such as frequent emergency department visits or high hospital readmission rates. Clinical integration attends to the core business of the system and can (and should) be the differentiating, value-added factor. It involves bringing roles, processes, resources, and services together to manage effectively the health and illness needs of individual patients and patient populations.

As a process that brings an integrated system together in a clinically functional and operational way, case management is a flexible and dynamic approach to managing the care of individual patients and patient populations. Comprehensive integrated systems are an ideal way to operationalize the concept of continuum of care; case management is continuum and episode-focused strategy to manage both clinical and cost outcomes. Because of these factors, there is universal recognition of the need for a systemwide case management process within integrated systems (Coile, 1995; Conrad, 1993; Fowler & Stokes, 1996). This chapter explores how case management fits into clinically integrated delivery systems and identifies key considerations for designing a case management practice for such a system.

Case Management As a Process to Manage Risk

Case management is one way to manage risk, and its design usually reflects the perceived real or potential risks encountered by the organization. The quality imperative to manage the continuum has always been a factor, especially for individuals at risk for poorer outcomes. However, the financial incentives are now more closely aligned with capitation and other managed care strategies. The mandate to manage the continuum and the episode is directly proportional to the degree of risk assumed for covered lives.

Because the nature of risk for various organizations differs, the focus of case management will also vary (see Figure 9.1). Risk extends along a continuum that has at one end the need to manage length of stay and cost per case in acute care settings within a Medicare DRG market, and at the other end the mandate to manage the health and wellness of covered lives in the community in a capitated market. Integrated delivery systems are often created to more effectively and aggressively pursue agreements with payers that involve higher degrees of risk, such as a degree of financial risk for clinical outcomes (Pelham, 1996).

Risk is rapidly changing in many markets. For example, Hudson (1997, p. 51) reports, "Last year, according to HCFA, an average of 80,000 Medicare recipients joined HMOs each month. Though HMO enrollees make up only 11 percent of Medicare beneficiaries, the figure is forecast to shoot skyward in the next decade." New types and higher levels of risk translate into diverse dimensions that must be effectively managed by a clinically integrated delivery system including the following:

- Illness → wellness
- Individual → populations
- Acute → chronic
- Point-of-service care → episode care → continuum care

Figure 9.1. Evolving Core of Case Management Roles.

Case Management Roles Follow Risk
(Clinical and Financial)

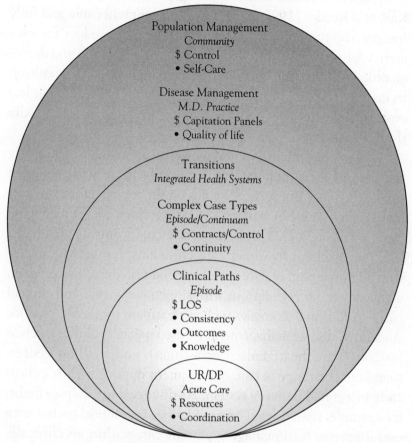

Population Management
Community
$ Control
• Self-Care

Disease Management
M.D. Practice
$ Capitation Panels
• Quality of life

Transitions
Integrated Health Systems

Complex Case Types
Episode/Continuum
$ Contracts/Control
• Continuity

Clinical Paths
Episode
$ LOS
• Consistency
• Outcomes
• Knowledge

UR/DP
Acute Care
$ Resources
• Coordination

Source: The Center for Case Management, 1997. Used with permission.

To deal with the diverse needs and issues before them, clinically integrated delivery systems must create a full and diverse array of points of care and care management strategies. As Kozma, Kaa, and Reeder (1997, p. 5) note, "A comprehensive and fully integrated continuum of care represents the new 'product' for integrated delivery networks. With the right number, mix, and demographic locations, the integrated delivery network is in a position to manage the care of its members across that continuum at less cost, with greater continuity and uniformity, and over markedly shorter wait times."

Case management is a very powerful approach to managing the care of focus populations, especially those with complex needs who place intensive demands on the system. However, case management must be part of a broader framework for managing care (see Figure 9.2). This framework includes unit- or area-based care management by direct care clinicians, resource managers who align the plan of care with financial resources, and program management for populations with similar care needs and clinical paths. Additional strategies such as treatment protocols, practice guidelines, disease management, focused specialty clinics (such as for congestive heart failure or asthma), and wellness centers round out the range of care management options within a clinically integrated delivery system. As discussed in Chapter Eight, for example, system-level care guidelines (or clinical paths) are a useful approach to managing patient care within an clinically integrated delivery system, especially for those high-volume patient populations with reasonable homogeneity and predictability in their care needs.

Patients on clinical paths can usually be managed by the clinical staff, leaving those patients who do not fit (and probably will never fit) on a clinical path to be supported by case managers. However, without a full array of options for managing care, case management will become a high-cost service, and the full range of results will not be realized.

**Figure 9.2. The Relationship of
Various Strategies to Coordinated Care.**

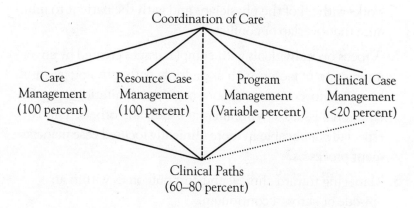

Coordination of Care

| Care Management (100 percent) | Resource Case Management (100 percent) | Program Management (Variable percent) | Clinical Case Management (<20 percent) |

Clinical Paths
(60–80 percent)

Source: The Center for Case Management, 1996. Used with permission.

Defining Case Management: An Integral Design Step

Defining case management is an important first step in creating a systemwide process, but definition is a complex process. Currently, the term *case management* can elicit confusion and disagreement, because, frequently, case management has been expected to address global and varied issues within an organization. Other sources of confusion are the diverse applications of case management, which speaks to the flexible nature of case management and to its evolution within health care.

Although the definitions and applications of case management seem diverse, a few key concepts are at the core of most of them:

1. Negotiating, procuring, and coordinating services and resources needed by patients and their families. Individuals needing case management often require services from multiple providers (clinical, social, and economic) that must be carefully sequenced and managed. For example, individuals with multiple pathophysiology will receive care from various

specialist physicians who may provide overlapping or conflicting prescriptions and recommendations. The case manager
works with all of the physicians and with the patient to minimize that overlap or conflict.

2. A focus on individuals with complex issues created by an
   interaction of factors such as multiple pathophysiology, insuf-
   ficient socioeconomic support, cognitive limitations, psycho-
   emotional issues, environmental issues, and others. This is
   especially applicable in more clinically focused case management processes.

3. Managing toward clinical and cost outcomes within an
   episode or across a continuum.

4. Using a clinical or scientific reasoning process to address
   patient and family needs (assessment, goal setting, plan
   implementation, evaluation, and revision).

5. Advocating for the needs of patients and their families.

6. Integrating and potentiating the contributions of various disciplines, resources, services, and sites.

The concepts of episode- and continuum-based management of
patient care are important, especially within an integrated delivery
system. Episode and continuum are distinct entities because strategies for managing each will be different. Episode-based issues have
a beginning and an end; continuum-based issues have a beginning,
but the end is typically death. Chronic illnesses are examples of
continuum-based issues because, although they may be well managed, they are an ongoing part of the individual's life. Individuals
with chronic illnesses have a particular need for effective care management because of the costs associated with their care over time.
This is especially true of costs related to recidivism, specifically the
causes of recidivism that can be decreased or eliminated.

Capitation has refocused attention on the need to manage
episode and continuum issues effectively in order to lower the intensity of services needed and thus the related costs. The applica-

tion of case management to continuum-focused issues usually results in long-term involvement with selected individuals, often extending over years, to support them at the lowest appropriate level of service intensity.

Definitions are also closely associated with desired outcomes for case management within the sponsoring entity. Case management, like clinically integrated delivery systems, is a means, not an end. The desired outcomes of case management are related to the risk levels noted earlier. The ultimate goal of case management, particularly in capitated markets, is to support individuals and their families at their highest level of functionality, comfort, and independence while at the lowest, most appropriate level of service.

Bringing Case Management and Clinical Integration Together

When the ink dries on the agreement creating an IDS, entities within the new organization often have some form of case management in place. And each entity is likely to have a vested interest in *its* approach to case management. As previously noted, varied approaches to case management grow out of organization-specific issues and risks. In addition, each site may serve very different sections of the catchment area. It is no wonder that case management (and clinical integration mechanisms in general) often end up at the center of a political maelstrom, with each site building a case for its own processes. The real work begins at this point. The goal is to bring the various approaches together into a coherent, consistent process that will be effective for the system, while building positive relationships among the entities. As Fowler and Stokes (1996, p. 65) suggest, "Systems with multiprovider sites and multiple levels of care should be well positioned to offer one-stop shopping. MCOs have shown high interest in this concept to reduce costs and have better leverage over quality. However, for this to happen some form of standardization and integration of case management systems must be in place. Without it, multiprovider groups with multiple levels of care do not offer any real advantage in the marketplace."

The Administrator's Role

For this to happen, administrators at the system level must identify when clinical integration design will begin, what is the time line for creating the first design phase, and who will be accountable for leading the design effort. In addition, the decision makers related to case management and other aspects of clinical integration must be identified. Without these elements in place, the clinical integration process, including the development of systemwide case management, will most likely suffer a series of false starts, to the intense frustration of all involved and to the detriment of the system's ability to effectively manage its core business.

Stages of Case Management Integration

The integration of case management, like other integration processes, typically moves through three stages:

1. Each setting within the system has its own roles, processes, systems, and structures.
2. Common definitions and expected outcomes emerge, although management of the process is still largely at the local levels.
3. Case management and other coordination processes become an integrated service that operates centrally at the system level, serving the needs of the entire system and its component parts.

The speed with which an integrated system moves through the stages is related to current and changing risks. For example, an integrated system may be composed of organizations that have not previously managed capitated contracts. When one of the first steps of the newly integrated organization is successfully negotiating a large capitated contract, the need for clinical integration becomes more intense. Specifically, it is suggested that when an organization experiences a managed care penetration of more than 30 percent for the population under 65 years of age or penetration in a Medicare risk population of 15 percent, there is readiness to move to a standardized and integrated case management system (Fowler & Stokes, 1996). This is an important indicator to monitor while creating a systemwide case management process within an IDS.

Assessing the Environment As a Foundation for Process Design

Moving from stage one to stage three requires concentrated effort, commitment, communication, persistence, and patience. It also requires a plan and a broad understanding of the environment in which the clinically integrated delivery system is emerging. The process begins with assessment of the current status of the environment and projections regarding future trends.

Multiple points must be assessed for a comprehensive understanding of the environment. They can be broadly categorized into those related to the system, the community, and the current level of care coordination within the integrated system. Examples follow of assessment points for each category.

About the system:

- To what extent is the system truly integrated? It is a loose affiliation or a full asset merger of various entities?

  At what stage is the integration of the administrative and financial components of the system?

- Is there an insurance product within the system?

- What is the nature and quality of the relationship between the integrated system and physicians within the community, both individual practitioners and group practices? What is the nature and level of risk assumed by the physicians?

- Is there clarity about who will have accountability for creating a system-level case management process and other clinical integration mechanisms? Have the decision makers been identified?

- Which risks are currently being managed by the system? What are the projections for future risks and the anticipated timetable for the change? To what extent is there managed care penetration within the region? For which populations? How is that likely to change in the near future?

- What are the high-volume and high-cost case types within each of the component entities and the integrated system as a whole?

  Is there an integrated information system? If so, which information is integrated (such as only financial or clinical or both)?

  What is the profile of populations served by each of the system entities? How are they alike? How do they differ?

  Which barriers prevent an integrated clinical process, including case management? How can they be addressed?

About the environment in which the integrated system exists:

- What are the needs and characteristics of the patients served by the system (demographics, risk factors, and so on)?

  What are the characteristics of the environment (including geographical size, urban or rural setting, physician members, and so on)?

- What is the current level of health within the community served by the integrated system? What are the most frequently seen risk factors in the community, including those related to health, social, economic, and environmental aspects?

- What is currently available to manage individuals and populations along a continuum, including prevention, wellness support and health maintenance, screening, primary care, urgent care, tertiary care, terminal care, long-term care, rehabilitation, respite care? How are gaps being addressed?
- What resources currently exist within the environment? (Consider formal, structured resources such as agencies and services, along with informal resources such as volunteer services.)
- What are the plans for addressing identified gaps in service within the community?

About the current status of clinical coordination within the system components:

- Which processes are in place to manage clinical and cost aspects of patient care? What are their strengths? Which outcomes are being measured? What is the assessment of the effectiveness of those processes on improving outcomes? Where do the processes need to be improved?
- What are the current staffing levels related to care management processes? What are the departmental structures?

    To what extent is there continuum management versus point-of-service management?

The time spent in gathering and analyzing this information is an essential foundation for the next phase, creating the design. Each element is influential in how care must be managed at both the individual and system levels. For example, if the IDS is at the stage where there is administrative but not financial integration, systemwide case management may not be an urgent priority. Timing is crucial in creating a systemwide case management process, and the design stage goes more smoothly the more incentives are aligned.

Support Structures for Case Management
in Integrated Systems

In addition to moving toward case management, it is important to establish administrative structures and systems that will functionally unite the various entities and to develop roles and processes to support patient care management. Internally and externally, the integrated system must be perceived as a unity. As Chapter Seven presented, an enterprisewide information system is a powerful integrative mechanism, but most IDS will not have this in place immediately; consequently, strategies must be invented for both the transition period and the long-term outcome. For example, patient information, including patient record numbers, must be transferable between and among care sites. Creating a methodology for systemwide patient record numbers is extremely complex process and evolves over time; it therefore must be initiated early.

Other processes must be centralized within the integrated system to support continuum-based, multisite care. Ultimate support of the integrated system at the clinical and administrative levels includes an enterprisewide patient resource center. Such a center is "housed" at the corporate level of the structure and performs various functions:

1. It admits all clients to the integrated system from all service points.

2. Collects and maintains uniform data regarding the patient (including payer information).

3. Assigns a patient identification number that is used with all service points within the system.

4. Responds to information needs from patients, providers and payers, on a twenty-four-hour, seven-day basis as needed.

5. Completes preadmission and precertification processes and communicates with the payer for routine processing. Based on the response and the situation, the patient or payer can then be referred to an internal resource consultant.

6. Maintains a current list of available sites for care within the community, including long-term care beds, rehabilitation beds, and so on.

The patient resource center model is under design at Veterans' Memorial Medical Center in Meriden, Connecticut. It creates the "one-stop shopping" that is in great demand and provides consistent, current information upon which decisions can be made. The value of this center is enhanced if it also provides triaging of patient needs to various resources, including community resources, urgent care, physician referral, case management, "Ask-a-Nurse," and so on. Additional value is added if the center is a source of current information for health-related resources in the community. This type of center is a major resource and support to the case management process within the system.

Creating the Case Management Design

As a transitional step toward the creation of a design, the system-level administrative team should develop a broad description of elements of case management, including (1) specifically formulated goals for case management, (2) parameters for case management design (such as focus on acute versus community care or the need to align the case management practice with physician groups), (3) current and projected levels of risk to be managed, (4) resources available, (5) degree of desired integration, and (6) time frame. This articulation needs to be clear enough to enable a group to begin the system-level process yet flexible enough to permit findings by the group to truly shape that process.

The Design Team

A design team is an efficient vehicle for creating the case management process and structure for the integrated system and should be convened as soon as indicated on the clinical integration time line.

The design team brings together representatives from the case management processes in each site within the system, as well as those with an actual or potential interest. Membership generally includes social workers, nurses, quality management, utilization management, discharge planning, and administrators. At various points, members may also be needed from affiliated entities. For instance, if the integrated system does not include a formal relationship with the physician practices, it is wise to include representatives from that sector on the team. In addition to the description of the product by the administrative staff, the design team will need other resources:

1. A facilitator who focuses on the group process.

2. Access to the authorized decision makers on a regular basis for exchange of ideas and feedback about direction the team is taking.

3. Secretarial support (to arrange meetings, type minutes, and so on).

4. Clear direction to the managers of the various team members that participation in the team activities is a system-level priority, and time must be allocated for that purpose.

Elements of Case Management Functionality

The team works toward maximum functionality of case management within the clinically integrated delivery system. Functionality is related to the following features:

1. A core definition of case management that is sufficiently flexible to accommodate various needs and issues.

2. Measurable goals for the case management process, based on the broad goals established by the administrative team.

3. Well-defined focus populations for case management. Because case management creates additional roles within the system,

it is crucial to identify those patients who are most in need of those services.

4. Case managers who are positioned along all points of the continuum.

5. Role descriptions for the case managers that are realistic and differentiated from other roles within the organization.

6. A clearly defined reporting structure within the integrated system, including clarity about where the budget for case management will be managed (salaries, benefits, supplies, and so on).

7. A structure for how the case management practice will be organized and managed.

8. Referral, screening, and triaging criteria and processes for accepting patients into the case management practice from anywhere within the IDS. These criteria often reflect the need to case manage individuals who (1) experience frequent readmissions (to acute care, emergency departments, and other areas of high-intensity service) and (2) have poly-pharmacy, multiple pathophysiology, multiple physicians, marginal or ineffective socioeconomic situations, and cognitive or emotional issues influencing their ability for self-management.

9. A marketing plan to strategically inform the various constituents about the service.

10. A process by which case management outcomes are assessed regularly, using concrete and agreed upon measures, with the results shared among all the entities within the IDS.

Cultural Integration

Anticipate "tugs of culture" as the team comes together. Here are basic approaches to fast-tracking the process by the design team that may help expedite the process:

1. Recognize different approaches and cultures but do not get mired in them.

2. Regularly refocus on the desired outcome: to create a dynamic system for the effective and efficient management of patient care across the various entities of the clinically integrated delivery system.

3. Acknowledge that more than one approach to case management will be needed within a clinically integrated delivery system. Look toward knitting these approaches into a smooth process.

4. Know when to seek additional guidance, consultation, and assistance, and obtain it in a timely way.

5. Convene the team for more than one hour at a time. Block out three- or four-hour periods to facilitate continued progress. Creating a case management process requires continuity of thought and the opportunity to break through barriers. One hour meetings do not effectively provide that opportunity.

6. Identify a facilitator for the design team that can productively channel the group process and challenge the group to focus on case management for the system.

Case Management Dimensions in an Integrated System

Because the team is developing the case management process for the integrated system, its members must consider many dimensions: management both of individual patients and of populations; financial and clinical management; focus on health and wellness as well as managing illness; and point-of-service management and episode and continuum management of care. The need to manage both populations and individuals is underscored by Conrad (1993, p. 492), who asserts that "the essence of a system is the ability to "aggregate up" individual level care coordination and clinical processes into a system-level capacity to plan, deliver, monitor, and adjust the structures and strategies for coordinating the care of populations over time. The coordination of care for individual patients is a necessary, but not sufficient, condition to realizing system level clinical integration." Given these dimensions, more than one approach to case management will be needed. Examples of such approaches are described in the next sections.

Broad Spectrum Case Management Application

Within a clinically integrated delivery system, the case management practice must respond to the needs of multiple constituencies and situations. As noted earlier, this means that case managers work with clients in all sites throughout the continuum. As the penetration of capitation increases, the size and breadth of the case management practice will also expand.

Within the practice, some case managers will attend to the needs of patients with complex situations and support their transition throughout multiple points within an inpatient setting. Others will focus on responding to the complex financial situations that emerge for a subset of patients and interact closely with the patient resource center.

Still others will be based in the community, responding to referrals from inpatient staff and case managers, physician office staff, and other sources regarding the need to coordinate the care of patients in diverse sites, such as their homes, nursing homes, and rehabilitation centers. It is prudent to position some case managers in the offices of selected physician group practices. Others will work with individuals within large employers in the area, especially those with whom there is a strong relationship or a bundled contract.

Other case managers may have a specialized practice, focusing on populations that are simultaneously high volume and high cost. The cardiopulmonary and neonatal populations are examples of patients that often need specialized case management. There will also be a cadre of case managers who will follow selected clients throughout the entire continuum, coordinating their care in all sites. Transition among the members of the case management network is a crucial process that must be clearly defined. Case management becomes the web, linking the various sites within and external to the clinically integrated delivery system. This web must be strong enough and sufficiently widespread to address far reaching issues.

Although some individuals may only need temporary (or episodic) support from case managers, others may require long-term case management. These are often the chronically ill who demonstrate difficulty in managing their disease process and its treatment (such as individuals struggling with congestive heart failure, diabetes, or chronic destructive pulmonary disease). Readmission to acute care (or an increase in the intensity of services needed) is a warning signal for this population. In this situation, case management may be needed for the life of the individual, extending over several years with a goal of reducing acute care admissions. This is accomplished through implementing earlier detection and management of issues, as well as supporting individual patients in their ability for self-management. Case management is a long-term commitment and is based on loss avoidance rather than revenue generation.

Guidelines for the case management practice need to be discussed and agreed on as the practice forms. The differentiation between and among services is a critical factor for efficiency and success. For example, some case managers may provide services in clients' homes, which necessitates clarification of the interface with and differentiation from home health. Vigilance and ongoing communication are required to avoid duplication, and gaps in service.

The Group Practice Model

The group practice structure is an effective approach to managing case management in an IDS, especially those with multiple case managers and care sites. Group practice membership includes *all* individuals within the integrated system with the role responsibility of case manager. Group practices address issues such as consistency of practice, triage, screening criteria and procedures, process and outcome quality assessment and management, peer consultation, and ongoing education for the case managers. Group practice members identify how case management services will be provided without interruption in the planned and unplanned absences of case managers.

This model requires a central site for receiving referral calls, faxes, and e-mail. The practice must also establish how the referrals will receive a timely response and how patients and clients will be responded to in a timely manner. A case management group practice creates a self-directed work team and results in a more consistent application of case management throughout the system.

Beyond Implementation

Completion of the first phase of design and implementation is not the end of the journey. Case management design must be revisited at regular intervals to respond to the constantly changing market in which the integrated system functions. Periodic reassessment is needed to ensure that case management continues to meet the changing needs of the patients and the organization. Such reviews must be built into the process and attended to by the administrative staff.

Conclusion

The goals and function of clinically integrated delivery systems and case management are synergistic in many ways: continuum-and episode-focused management of patient care; efficiency and effectiveness; achievement of clinical and cost outcomes; and management of both individuals and populations of patients. Thus, case management is a key mechanism for clinical integration in an IDS.

In turn, case management is likely to be more successful within a structured IDS, due to the increased breadth of services and resources available. Although it is a powerful approach to managing care, case management is not the only available process. Effective, clinically integrated delivery systems will position case management appropriately within a panel of approaches and focus it to meet specific client and system needs. In this way, the IDS can truly provide coordinated, comprehensive care to those it serves.

References

Coile, R. C. (1995). Integration, capitation and managed care: Transformation of nursing for 21st-century health care. *Advanced Practice Nursing Quarterly, 1*(2), 77–84.

Conrad, D. (1993). Coordinating patient care services in regional health systems: The challenge of clinical integration. *Hospital and Health Services Administration, 38*(4), 491–508.

Fowler, F., & Stokes, J. (1996). Case management for multiprovider systems. *Case Manager, 7*(5), 63–69.

Hudson, T. (1997). Senior surge: Are you ready? *Hospitals and Health Networks, 71*(7), 51–56.

Kozma, C., Kaa, K., & Reeder, C. (1997). A model for comprehensive disease state management. *Journal of Outcomes Management, 4*(1), 4–8.

Pelham, J. (1996). Talk show. *Hospitals and Health Networks, 70*(14), 34–42.

Chapter Ten

Systemwide CQI and Education as an Integrative Engine

Bonita Ann Pilon

Three mechanisms to facilitate clinical integration have been presented in this part of the book: information systems, clinical paths and CareMaps, and case management. This chapter describes and interrelates three additional mechanisms that can greatly enhance clinical integration: (1) continuous quality improvement and total quality management (CQI and TQM), (2) outcomes measurement and management, and (3) education. These components have a synergistic effect in improving the health of populations. Effecting these strategies in an integrated delivery system requires unwavering commitment from all involved, particularly from senior leadership. This special responsibility of agency and system leaders is highlighted in this chapter.

Clinical Quality Improvement and Outcomes Measurement and Management

Creating a culture of clinical quality has long been a stated goal of health care providers, but methods for achieving quality have varied considerably until this decade. Since 1990, the methods and philosophies of Deming and others have increasingly permeated the U.S. health care workplace. Most notably, the Joint Commission on Accreditation of Healthcare Organizations (JCAHO) has made performance improvement the basis for its surveys of hospitals and other agencies beginning in 1994. Gone is the sole reliance on inspection of retrospective data to determine the quality of the organization's performance. Instead, the JCAHO looks for evidence of using data to improve quality in clinical systems and in those processes that support the delivery of patient care.

Within the managed care industry, the National Committee on Quality Assurance (NCQA) developed the HEDIS tool (Health Plan Employer Data and Information Set) to measure the quality of services within the health plan. Version 3.0, released in July 1996, measures plan performance on a number of dimensions: effectiveness of care, access to and availability of care, satisfaction with the experience of care, health plan stability, use of services, cost of care, and informed health choices. The tool measures both process (such as emphasis on smoking cessation) and outcome data (such as prevention of heart disease), as well as mortality rates after heart surgery (to treat heart disease). NCQA accreditation, though still largely voluntary, is growing in importance as a competitive advantage for managed care companies. According to the NCQA, HEDIS has been implemented by more than 330 plans and has become the national standard for measuring and comparing health plan performance (NCQA, 1996).

Outcomes Measurement

As the emphasis on quality improvement continues to increase, providers and health services researchers have turned to outcomes as the most important measure of the quality of care. Melum (1995, p. 6) defines *outcomes measurement* as "a structured system to evaluate health outcomes in a way that permits inferences about the relationship between health services and health outcomes. It includes collection of patient-based measures of outcome such as functional status and well-being, measures of clinical and other factors believed to be predictive of outcome, and patient-specific outcomes measures." Categories of outcomes related to health of individuals and populations include mortality, incidence of chronic disease, functional status, well-being, satisfaction, cost, and traditional clinical parameters such as blood pressure, blood sugar level, cholesterol level, and so on.

Outcomes measurement is an important first step. However, measurement without follow-up action will not improve the health of the population from which the measures were obtained. Davies and her colleagues have argued that managing outcomes is the means by which health outcomes can be improved (Davies, Doyle, Lansky, Rutt, Stevic, & Doyle, 1994). They defined *outcomes management* as "the use of information and knowledge gained from outcomes monitoring to achieve optimal patient outcomes, through improved clinical decision making and service delivery" (p. 9).

CQI and Outcomes Management

Continuous quality improvement and outcomes management share at least four common commitments: (1) meeting customer needs and expectations; (2) measuring quality; (3) increasing knowledge of how processes affect outcomes; and (4) continuously improving health care quality (Melum, 1995). Each approach is limited when taken alone, however. CQI is often focused on process rather than results. Outcomes management has produced good data on what the outcomes are, but may struggle with how to improve the outcomes once they are known. Integration of these approaches is a powerful unifying strategy for clinical systems.

In his classic article, Reinertsen (1993) argues for such integration when describing the health care system as a sailboat adrift at sea in a dense fog, with neither a compass nor a rudder. In addition, the ship has a limited fuel supply (shrinking health care resources). It does have a desired direction (that is, the best possible health results for patients). Reinertsen questions which would benefit the captain of the ship more: a compass or a rudder? From his perspective, CQI is like a rudder: it promotes reduction in variation, waste, and unnecessary complexity of processes and systems. With such a rudder, the boat could sail efficiently in a desired direction. The problem is, the captain doesn't know in which direction to sail. Outcomes measurement and management is the compass. The data on outcomes clarify the direction in which to sail to obtain the desired results. But without a rudder (CQI), the ship cannot steer itself efficiently in any direction. Reinertsen asserts that the sailboat would be out of control and widely variable—much like our current health care system. The ship (U.S. health care), he says, needs both a rudder and a compass. Neither is sufficient by itself. Table 10.1 illustrates Reinertsen's point.

Case Examples. Utilizing both the compass and the rudder— a synergistic approach—to improve health status can serve to unify the efforts of diverse professionals across complex hospitals and in the community. Consider the following:

The orthopedic service in a large community medical center de-cided to use selected questions from the SF–36[1] and TyPE[2] indica-tor tools to survey their joint replacement patients before surgery (to obtain baseline data), and at six months after surgery. Data are obtained by face-to-face interview and by telephone, conducted by a registered nurse. Quarterly reports are presented at the orthopedic medical staff division meetings, comparing the results of the pre-and postsurgery measures for their patient population. Discussion of the data-based results of their work allows physicians and other clinical staff to monitor how well patients fare over time. Run charts or con-trol charts may be used to depict visually the trends in functional

Table 10.1. The Compass and the Rudder.

	Outcomes Management: The Compass	Continuous Quality Improvement: The Rudder
Aim	Defines system goals	Leads to reduction in variation and com-plexity in processes
Timing	Long term (months, years, decades)	Short term (days, weeks, months)
Measurement	Patient-reported outcomes	Key quality characteristics

Source: Adapted from Reinertsen, 1993, p. 6.

outcomes across the population. Bar charts may be used to demon-strate the amount of improvement postsurgery.

Through such monitoring, the team is able to focus its improve-ment efforts on specific processes, such as physical therapy regimens, timing of interventions, timeliness of transfer to rehabilitation facil-ities, and pain control. Cohorts may be compared, such as those patients who underwent physical therapy at home versus those who were admitted for short-term stays in rehab units. If significant dif-ferences are detected, those clinical agencies are included in any improvement efforts.

By combining both outcomes measurement and continuous improvement methods, the clinical team in this example integrates care effectively within its own complex institution and works with other components across their integrated network. The focus on data and sound methods for improvement create a common lan-guage and purpose for all clinicians involved in the care of this pop-ulation. Discussions take place based on data rather than on finger pointing. Clinicians in acute care can analyze the long-term results of their interventions and improve them.

The synergy of continuous improvement and outcomes mea-surement and management can also be employed effectively when diverse agencies are contemplating integration. Employing such an approach from the beginning of the integration dialogue can facil-itate meaningful discussion and action planning, as the following scenario illustrates:

A group of twenty-three independent community agencies serving the elderly, with diverse sponsorship ranging from philanthropy to government subsidy, formed a voluntary network. Although the agency representatives held regular meetings, there was little real communication among them with regard to services delivered or coordination of services for at-risk clients. Recognizing that their attempts at horizontal integration were not successful, they em-ployed an outside consultant in case management. After an initial assessment, the consultant convened the group leaders in order to reach consensus on four key questions:

1. Who is the customer? (Determine who the target population is and define criteria for inclusion and exclusion.)

2. What is the aim? (Identify why these agencies desire to work together in the network.)

3. What are the processes? (Describe what the perfect case management system would look like.)

4. What are the desired outcomes? (Specify what will be measured.)

Three small groups were convened to answer the questions, led by a group facilitator. In a half-day session, the network agencies reached consensus on the aim, clarified the customer, designed a series of key processes, and defined the outcome measures.

In this case, continuous improvement techniques were used to build the network, and outcome measures were agreed upon before services were initiated. This approach to integration diffused "turf" issues by effectively engaging the expertise of all member agencies, again focused on the customer. By defining outcomes before the integration began, data can be monitored from the onset. These data will continue to focus future discussion on the customer so that improvements can be made.

Use of CareMaps. Another example of using CQI and outcomes management as an integration tool incorporates CareMaps for managing for an episode of illness that encompasses more than one care venue. Stroke treatment and rehabilitation typically occur across at least two sites: acute care and a rehabilitation unit or facility. Creating and using stroke CareMaps puts CQI at the bedside, as they are designed to streamline care processes and eliminate unnecessary variations in practice. Evaluating the outcomes of the care regimen embodied in the map leads to opportunities for outcomes management: achievement of optimal patient outcomes through improved clinical decision making and service delivery. Outcome analysis informs the clinical team about the success of their efforts; continuous improvement methods provide the tools to identify and improve actual clinical and support system processes. After the processes are improved, outcomes are measured again. The integrated delivery system thus monitors progress in improving the health status of the population of stroke patients it serves.

Benchmarking. Another strategy helpful for integration of clinical systems is the use of benchmark data for comparing results from other populations (of patients, providers, or both), and for motivating diverse agencies and providers to begin to work in concert to improve clinical and financial outcomes. For example, *physician profiling*—blind comparisons of cost per case (using severity-adjusted DRGs) among a group of physicians and against state or national data—provides the clinician with objective results of his or her work over time. Periodic, data-driven feedback (hallmarks of continuous improvement) assist diverse clinicians throughout the system to decrease wide variations in practice (also a hallmark of continuous quality improvement). Severity-adjusted tools are key to the credibility of the data and the validity of the resulting comparisons.

In summary, the health of populations cared for by emerging integrated delivery systems is best served when the provider network understands and embraces the principles and methods of continuous quality improvement. In addition, the network must be committed to measuring the results of its work: clinical outcomes. These outcomes should encompass far more than the traditional negative measures, such as mortality and morbidity. Patient-centered outcomes—functional status, ability to work, role function, quality of life—are critical indicators for the effectiveness of the health care delivery system. When integrated providers evaluate these data, their efforts to improve the quality of care can be more precisely focused to achieve desired results. The reciprocal relationship between improvement of care processes and measurement of patient outcomes is powerful and never-ending.

Role of Education in Clinical Integration

Closely linked to continuous quality improvement and outcomes management, education is a mechanism that can be very effective in helping to create and sustain clinical integration within an integrated delivery system. Education is discussed here in the broadest context—patient and family education, provider education, and leadership education within the clinical enterprise.

Vital and Expanding Role of Consumers

Consumers demand an increased role in treatment decisions and choice of provider. The growth of point-of-service HMO products in this decade acknowledges consumers' wishes for choice of provider, even in the face of increased managed care penetration in regional markets. Living wills, durable medical powers of attorney, and the Patients' Bill of Rights clearly indicate the increased voice of the customer in treatment decisions.

In addition to these obvious shifts in the traditional health care paradigm, more subtle changes are occurring at the provider-patient interface. Patients and their families are being educated and empowered to self-manage their chronic illnesses. Consider just a few examples: in-home glucose monitoring by diabetics; in-home blood pressure monitoring and graphing of results on a run chart by the patient or family; family-managed peritoneal dialysis at home; epidural pain medication dosing by family members; and monitoring of congestive heart failure patients' fluid loads and functional status by the patient or family.

These examples illustrate a fundamental premise of clinical integration that may be overlooked: integrated delivery systems are more than a network of agencies, clinical providers, and insurers. They must also actively incorporate patients and their families if they wish to affect the health of populations. The most effective strategy for engaging patients in self-management is education through an ongoing supportive, trustful relationship with the provider network. As care for chronic illness moves to the home and community, the imperative for teaching patients and families to self-manage their symptoms will increase exponentially. Visionary integrated delivery system leaders will recognize this trend and build programs that address the need for comprehensive patient and family education.

Clinical Practice Guidelines

For providers, the synergy among continuous quality improvement, outcomes management, and education is readily apparent in the clinical practice guidelines, which continue to be developed and disseminated. Used by providers systemwide, the guidelines attempt to reduce wide variability in treatment regimens among providers. Such guidelines are developed by the providers themselves within the network or may be adopted in whole or in part from national or regional consensus documents.

The Agency for Health Care Policy and Research (AHCPR) has funded fourteen PORTs (Patient Oriented Research Teams) since 1989, looking specifically at the data-supported outcomes for targeted conditions, using specific interventions. The conditions selected include those about which data are available or can be obtained (*1997 Medical Outcomes and Guidelines Sourcebook*) and those that demonstrate a wide variation in clinical practice intervention, affect large volumes of people, and involve expensive treatment. Conditions such as hip fracture, pneumonia, back pain, ischemic heart disease, diabetes, and stroke prevention have been studied. A second generation of PORTs, called PORT IIs, are now working to extend the work of the original studies.

Findings from the PORTs have been used to develop clinical practice guidelines for physicians and other providers. These guidelines educate providers regarding effective treatment, demonstrated to achieve optimal patient outcomes. Through this synergy of outcome research, education, and continuous improvement of clinical processes, the health of the population can be improved.

AHCPR-sponsored research has been the foundation of other educational efforts. In addition to the clinical practice guidelines for clinicians, by the end of 1996 the agency also had produced and disseminated nineteen guidelines for the general public (*1997 Medical Outcomes and Guidelines Sourcebook*). These include publications targeting otitis media, cancer pain, low back pain, and urinary incontinence. This education initiative is data-based (from the PORT studies) and aims to improve the health status of the population by increasing their self-care management skills and knowledge. (More information about clinician and consumer guidelines can be obtained from the AHCPR's World Wide Web site: [www.ahcpr.gov].)

Role of Senior Leadership: CQI, Outcomes Management, and Education

Effective clinical integration, built on continuous quality improvement methods, outcome management, and education of patients and providers, cannot happen without the active commitment of senior leaders. Actions speak louder than words—a systemwide culture of clinical quality cannot be delegated to a quality manager who is buried deep in the organization, distant from the CEO and board, and lacking sufficient power to change behavior. Executives who talk about quality in their organizations but fail to demonstrate their personal involvement and commitment are abdicating their leadership responsibilities. Compare these two case examples:

The newly promoted CEO of a large (over 500-bed), financially successful community medical center spoke often about the hospital's "caring" and its quality reputation. The executive team actively sought and accomplished integrated delivery system growth through acquisitions, mergers, and partnerships. The pursuit of quality within this system was delegated four layers down the organization, with the CEO's admonition to "just make me look good." The newly employed quality team advised senior leadership of serious gaps in the performance improvement plan, which would impact JCAHO accreditation. Numerous recommendations were made to close those gaps, including special education sessions for senior administrative and medical staff leaders to create a common language and knowledge base for sustaining a culture of quality improvement.

The CEO attended less than one hour of a twelve-hour focused training initiative on quality. Several executive-level vice presidents were also not committed to CQI and had been undermining JCAHO accreditation preparation as efforts to meet "unreasonable requirements." (This hospital had last been surveyed in 1993, before the performance improvement emphasis was fully implemented.) The CEO's failure to make quality training a personal and leadership priority sent a strong message to subordinates: they too could dismiss its importance.

The hospital subsequently requested a delay in its accreditation visit (at the urging of the quality team) and underwent a one-day extension survey. During that one-day cursory process, twelve Type I recommendations were given. (Type I recommendations occur when the hospital has not met JCAHO's standards in a specific area, such as timely completion of medical records. Each Type I must be corrected and documented within a short period of time. If the survey team finds unsafe conditions or a pattern of substandard conditions, the hospital may lose its accreditation status. Many payers, including Medicare and Medicaid, will not approve payment to hospitals that are not accredited.) A full survey was scheduled for nine months later. Senior leadership has taken note of the accreditation results but continues to focus efforts to improve by hiring a series of consultants to advise on "programs." The CEO and several key members of the executive team do not yet "walk the talk" of quality improvement and outcomes management. There has been little use of CQI, outcomes management, and targeted education initiatives to achieve clinical integration. Although the hospital considers itself at the hub of an integrated delivery system, it remains a collection of agencies, providers, and insurers connected only by financial arrangements and incentives.

Another hospital CEO took a very different approach. Quality improvement was made the top priority of the institution, starting in the executive office. Smaller in size, this agency lacked the internal resources to initiate a culture change to continuous improvement. After careful study, the executive team employed one consulting company, working closely with them over several years to integrate quality principles into the fabric of the organization. All senior leaders, led by the CEO, plus physician leaders went off-site to a series of quality education sessions. Performance improvement standards were developed and progress reports were made to the board. Commendation from the JCAHO accreditation process was seen as an intermediate goal for this organization. Over a five-year period, they met and exceeded their goal, by becoming the first health care industry recipient of the statewide quality award, meeting tough external review criteria.

These hospitals, both part of larger delivery systems, were led to very different results by their CEOs. Daniel Beckham, national director of consulting for Quorum Health Resources, gives this advice to health care CEOs:

I have been an ardent defender of American health care managers. I still believe that they have earned that defense. But I would also suggest that they ought to be very busy at work recrafting their organizations, and there are clearly places to start. First, drive out the dangerous and the uncommitted. Second, break down the functional and specialty walls. Third, demand standardization of work. Fourth, do all of these things with doctors, as well as the people who are on the hospital's payroll. For hospital and system CEOs, there ought to be personal priorities. They can't be fully delegated, nor can they be easily mandated. They require something else. It's called leadership [Beckham, 1993, p. 98].

Commitment Required for Success

CEOs and other senior leaders must understand and embrace the methods and principles of continuous improvement, integrated within an outcomes management approach, if they are to lead their organizations to effective clinical integration. Often such commitment begins with education targeted to senior executives. Learning organizations, according to Senge (1990), are continually learning and shedding their former mental models. Such work is begun and sustained by the CEO.

Once committed to clinical integration supported by CQI and outcomes management, senior leaders need to find effective ways to turn data into meaningful information. Data-based clinical improvement initiatives produce myriad actual and potential reports: which data are important to gather, and with whom should they be shared? It is the role of executive leadership to decide the cost benefit of data gathering, which includes assessment of the burden on caregivers and patients for data collection, the cost of analysts to create reports, and the cost of technology that supports complex databases. The key questions to be answered are, What is the cost of knowing, and what difference would it make if we did? Not every comparison adds value to the organization or system.

Once the organization reaches consensus on which data are to be collected, the reporting format and schedule can be determined. At the senior leadership level, including the board, the Value Compass approach is very useful in synthesizing clinical, outcomes, satisfaction, and cost and utilization data that clinicians, executives, and the board can use to make decision. Developed by Nelson and colleagues at Dartmouth (Nelson, Mohr, Batalden, & Plume, 1996; Nelson, Batalden, Plume, & Mohr, 1996), the Value Compass is a concise "dashboard" approach to integrated delivery systems and individual agencies (see Figure 10.1).

Figure 10.1. The Value Compass.

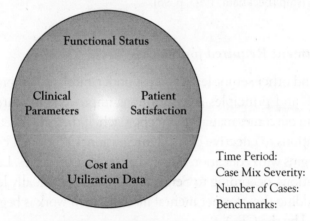

Time Period:
Case Mix Severity:
Number of Cases:
Benchmarks:

Source: Adapted from Batalden, Mohr, Nelson, & Plume, 1996; Nelson, Mohr, Batalden, & Plume, 1996; Nelson, Batalden, Plume, & Mohr, 1996; Mohr, Mahoney, Nelson, Batalden, & Plume, 1996.

The most important indicators for each category are highlighted within the compass, and summary data about the target population, including benchmarks, are displayed in the lower right-hand corner. For example, the cost or charges per case and average length of stay for the reporting period are displayed in the Cost and Utilization Data section. SF–36 scores or other outcomes data are displayed in the Functional Status area. Patient satisfaction scores are entered in the Patient Satisfaction area and clinical indicators, targeted for the specific diagnosis (such as infection rates for surgical diagnoses or blood sugar levels for diabetics) are found in the Clinical Parameters section. This tool helps the user to integrate and synthesize various types of data in order to discern how successful the health care system has been in achieving optimal levels of health for the targeted population. Both executives and providers can use this framework to judge the effectiveness of their efforts.

Role of the Governing Board

If the role of senior executives is to lead their organizations to a culture of clinical integration founded on quality improvement, outcomes management, and ongoing education, it is apparent then, that the role of the governing board is to hold CEOs accountable for accomplishing these objectives. Hospital boards, especially among the not-for-profit sector, have a rich history of community and religious service as their mission. While these values cannot be overlooked in the tumultuous and competitive health care market, boards cannot ignore clear imperatives to be active rather than passive in their service. Moving from a cottage industry, community service approach to a highly competitive, systemwide, quality-driven environment requires change at the board level.

New Knowledge and Skills

Traditional boards may include a majority of members with no health care background, which makes it difficult for them to evaluate the operation of the enterprise. Or boards may be composed of too many insiders from the institution itself or from other agencies within the same integrated delivery system. In both cases the board may be ill prepared or ill motivated to evaluate critically the agency's progress in quality improvement and outcomes management. Financial performance may remain the only objective measure on which the board judges the success of the system. Without a thorough understanding of and appreciation for the value of quality, governing boards can have too narrow a focus. Numerous examples from other industries have taught us that financial performance of a business is a function of the quality of the product or service, as much or more than the volume or price of goods sold. Health care boards are not yet as sophisticated in their approach to quality and outcomes.

Quality-focused health care agencies and systems will engage the governing board as a partner in creating a culture of clinical quality upon which to base clinical integration. The first step in this partnership is to educate the board about quality improvement methods and success stories within the industry. Board members should be familiar with the teachings of Deming and other quality leaders. Such educational initiatives take time; the integrated delivery system must invest in the development of the board. Several of Deming's fourteen points (1986, pp. 23–24) speak directly to the board:

- End the practice of awarding business on the basis of price tag alone.
- Teach and institute leadership.
- Drive out fear. Create trust. Create a climate for innovation.
- Eliminate management by objective. Instead, learn the capabilities of processes and how to improve them.
- Take action to accomplish the transformation.

Once familiar with the language, methods, and philosophy of CQI and outcomes management, the board should receive regular reports on key quality indicators, including patient outcomes. The Value Compass format is a succinct way of synthesizing data from numerous sources. Reports of this type on targeted product lines, such as cardiac surgery or women's health, should be regularly presented to the governing board. Educated and articulate board members will be active evaluators of the quality of the product produced by the integrated delivery system, as well as good stewards of the financial enterprise.

Conclusion

A shared culture of clinical quality improvement, targeted toward improving outcomes for patients, can be a powerful integrating mechanism for emerging health care delivery systems. Creating such a culture depends on an ongoing commitment to continuous learning and education throughout the network for both providers and patients. The catalyst for instigating this cultural transformation is senior leadership. Sustaining such an environment is the shared responsibility of senior leaders and the governing board. Health care organizations increasingly will be differentiated in the marketplace by the quality of the outcomes they produce. Quality and outcomes management are the rudder and the compass that allow us to sail our health care ship in the desired direction. The ship has already set sail.

Notes

1. The SF–36 was developed by Tarlov and colleagues as part of the Medical Outcomes Study (1989). Measures include general health perception, functional status, and well-being. Current versions include the Rand Corporation's thirty-six–item Health Status Survey and the Health Status Questionnaire (Version 2.0) from the Health Outcomes Institute. The latter contains three additional items that measure change in health and depression risk.

2. TyPE Indicator tools have been developed by the Health Outcomes Institute for specific conditions. These contain minimum sets of valid and reliable measures to be used in conjunction with SF–36 data to classify a patient's condition, interventions, and outcomes. These usually include clinical and laboratory data, treatment information, supplemental data on functional well-being, and symptoms.

References

The 1997 medical outcomes and guidelines sourcebook. (1996). New York: Faulkner and Gray.

Batalden, P. B., Mohr, J. J., Nelson, E. C., & Plume, S. K. (1996). Improving health care: Part 4. Concepts for improving any clinical process. *Joint Commission Journal on Quality Improvement, 22*(10), 651–659.

Beckham, J. D. (1993). Andrew's not-so-excellent adventure. *Healthcare Forum Journal, 36*(3), 90–94, 96, 98.

Davies, A. R., Doyle, M.A.T., Lansky, D., Rutt, W., Stevic, M. O., & Doyle, J. B. (1994). Outcomes assessment in clinical settings: A consensus statement on principles and best practices in project management. *Joint Commission Journal on Quality Improvement, 20*(1), 6–16.

Deming, W. E. (1986). *Out of the crisis*. Cambridge, MA: MIT Center for Advanced Engineering Study.

Melum, M. M. (1995). *Total quality outcomes management: A guide to integrating outcomes measurement and TQM to improve health.* Methuen, MA: GOAL/QPC.

Mohr, J. J., Mahoney, C. C., Nelson, E. C., Batalden, P. B., & Plume, S. K. (1996). Improving health care: Part 3. Clinical benchmarking for best patient care. *Joint Commission Journal on Quality Improvement, 22*(9), 599–616.

NCQA (National Committee on Quality Assurance). (1996). NCQA issues a draft of HEDIS 3.0. [http://www.ncqa.org/news/hedis3.0.htm].

Nelson, E.C., Batalden, P. B., Plume, S. K., & Mohr, J. J. (1996). Improving health care: Part 2. A clinical improvement worksheet and users' manual. *Joint Commission Journal on Quality Improvement, 22*(8), 531–548.

Nelson, E. C., Mohr, J. J., Batalden, P. B., & Plume, S. K. (1996). Improving health care: Part 1. The clinical value compass. *Joint Commission Journal on Quality Improvement, 22*(4), 243–258.

Reinertsen, J. L. (1993). Outcomes management and continuous quality improvement: The compass and the rudder. *Quality Review Bulletin, 19*(1), 5–7.

Senge, P. (1990). *The fifth discipline: The art and practice of the learning organization.* New York: Doubleday.

Tarlov, A. R., Ware, J. E., Greenfield, S., Nelson, E. C., Perrin, E., & Zubkoff, M. (1989). The medical outcomes study: An application of methods for monitoring the results of medical care. *Journal of the American Medical Association, 262,* 925–930.

Chapter Eleven

Common Themes and Concluding Thoughts

Mary Crabtree Tonges

Impelled by market-driven reforms, health care leaders are striving to combine isolated components of service into organized delivery systems. The central argument of this book is that these systems will fulfill their promise for providing quality care at a lower cost to the extent that their clinical services are tightly integrated. Our goal has been to illustrate mechanisms to achieve that end. This concluding chapter presents my summary of the book's themes and key points and suggestions for further research.

Theme One: The Changing Nature and Importance of Relationships

As health care restructures, relationships are changing at every level, from interorganizational to interpersonal. Yet the quality of these relationships is more important than ever. Consider the following examples:

- At the macro level, links between employers, purchasers, and providers are undergoing major changes as IDS decrease transaction costs and assume increased accountability for outcomes.
- In their relationships with each other, health organizations are shifting from being independent competitors to members of an integrated system, competing with other IDS.

- Hospitals are moving from interacting with individual patients during episodes of acute care to providing a full range of population-oriented health services to their communities.

- Physicians and hospitals must work together more closely than ever before, sharing common incentives for the first time. As Williams notes, success in these endeavors depends heavily on human relationships.

- At a micro level, clinicians are becoming increasingly more cognizant of their interdependence and the need for collaboration, communication, and trust. Henry and Anderson's joint leadership of their product line exemplifies this new spirit of cooperation.

- Finally, and perhaps most importantly, provider-patient relationships are changing as patients and families become more knowledgeable and active in managing their health.

In summary, many old, comfortable relationships have been lost, and new ones must be developed with other players. Trust and teamwork in these emerging relationships among clinicians, administrators, and clients are fundamental to the success of IDS.

Theme Two: The Need for Leadership

Many of the authors identify the importance of executive leadership, highlighting the leader's responsibility for articulating a clear vision of what the system is to become and guiding the cultural transformation required to achieve this goal. As one of the strongest proponents of this message, Pilon stresses the need for "unwavering commitment" from senior management, who must also be willing to "walk the talk" through highly visible and active participation. She brings the point home with powerful examples of different CEOs' approaches to these issues and the consequences for their organizations. Robertson also illustrates the central role the CEO at North Shore has played in developing the system and facilitating the creation and expansion of the path program.

Williams speaks to the need for CEO and board commitment to involving physicians in the growth of the enterprise, supported by a willingness to listen to and meet physicians' needs. Anderson also highlights the leadership responsibilities of physicians.

Jacobsen and Hill point out that care management automation will founder without leadership from an executive steering committee, and Bower makes similar points regarding the development of a systemwide case management program. Jacobsen and Hill also emphasize the importance of CEO- and board-level recognition of the need for a clinical information system to strengthen communication and continuity of care and approval of the necessary funding. Without top level commitment, manifested in active involvement and support, clinical integration will not happen.

Theme Three: Rewards and Risks of Information Technology

Jacobsen and Hill and others speak to both the promise and integrative potential of IT, and the challenges posed by complex, multiorganization entities. Their vision of information available "everywhere, every time, to everyone" can make seamless communication and continuity of care a reality. To use Ritter-Teitel's term, clinical reengineering projects, such as electronic medical record initiatives, are underway in IDS around the country. IT can also greatly enhance our ability to capture the data needed to measure outcomes of care and demonstrate value to outside reviewers. Equally, if not more importantly, decision-support systems for clinicians should move us from the realm of just increasing efficiency (doing the same things faster, cheaper) to improving effectiveness (better care processes and outcomes).

As anyone who uses a computer knows, informatics is a young science, and automation is frequently a difficult process. Problems of incompatibility, vaporware, glitches, crashes, and so on are often part our current reality, and the complexity of designing and installing systems multiplies as new organizations are added to the enterprise. Compounding these issues is the sensitivity of the information involved. Most people are probably more concerned about the confidentiality of their health records than their finances.

Nevertheless, Ummel (1997, p. 76) suggests that information technology is "arguably one of the most powerful continuum-building tools." Indeed, if culture is the most powerful integrator, IT may be a close second, and Jacobsen and Hill offer good advice for IDS striving to meet the challenge of actualizing this potential.

Theme Four: Multiple Approaches and Synergistic Effects

One of the key messages of this book is that multiple approaches to integrating care are needed. Just as a system is greater than the sum of its parts, a combination of mechanisms may create synergistic effects that yield incremental benefits over and above the effects of any one of them in isolation. This is also true at the level of individual mechanisms, such as clinical paths and CareMaps, which combine the complementary features of documentation by exception and variance analysis and management. As Henry describes, the whole package creates an effective path system.

Pilon clearly articulates the value of integrating continuous quality improvement, outcomes management, and education. Ritter-Teitel and Jacobsen and Hill suggest that intraorganizational care management mechanisms, such as clinical paths and case management, facilitate the development of both interorganizational mechanisms and clinical information systems. Williams's recommended approach for influencing physician behavior is also multifaceted.

Perhaps the most comprehensive example of synthesis is provided by Blouin, Kaplan, and Buturusis. Their spider diagram integrates all of the major topics of this book:

- Goals and vision (culture)
- Information systems

- Care management (paths and case management)
- Physician parternships and incentives
- Outcomes management (CQI)
- Core processes (product line structure)

IDS that harness the synergistic effects of these interrelated capabilities will create a powerful force for clinical integration.

In the first chapter, the effectiveness of a linear approach to integration was questioned. Turning again to Zander's ideas, she proposes that disease management (and, ultimately, health management) requires a broader approach than our traditional medical model, which tends to focus on specific organs and body systems (personal communication, 1997). As an alternative, she suggests that the form and function of IDS should model the human body, a quintessential integrated system. Using the body as the organizational metaphor suggests, for example, that administrative integration may be likened to the autonomic nervous system, in that essential elements (such as communication and finance systems) can be expected to function without conscious effort on the part of clinicians. Zander's approach would also require a more holistic definition of populations, perhaps along combinations of life stages and wellness or illness (such as the frail elderly and the nonfrail but cardiorespiratory compromised).

Theme Five: The Long View on Payback from Prevention

Several authors refer to interventions aimed at primary or secondary prevention and the time frames for such programs. Henry describes a smoking cessation initiative and a congestive heart failure clinic. Bower discusses case management for the chronically ill, and Pilon indicates that outcomes management occurs over a period of years or decades.

Building on the systems thinking approach introduced in Chapter Four, another system archetype can be used to illustrate the choices presented by our health care system and the nature of the expected payback from prevention. Figure 11.1 depicts the "shifting-the-burden" archetype (Senge, 1990). In this type of system, a problem is creating the symptom in the center. The top loop represents a knee-jerk response resulting in a symptomatic "solution," while the bottom loop represents an approach that addresses the actual cause of the problem.

Although a fundamental solution may take longer, as the delay in the bottom loop indicates, it will ultimately produce sustained improvement. Moreover, the symptomatic approach can create side effects that make the basic problem worse. As these side effects begin to snowball, it becomes increasingly difficult to implement the fundamental solution. The key principle for managing this type of situation is to avoid quick fixes and concentrate on the fundamental solution (Senge, 1990). This archetype provides a useful framework for analyzing basic problems within the health care industry and the likely outcomes of alternative responses.

Figure 11.1. Shifting the Burden.

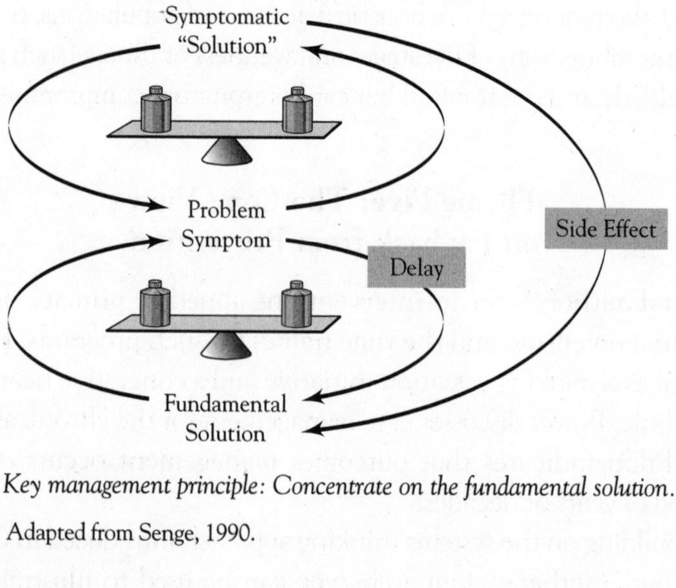

Key management principle: Concentrate on the fundamental solution.

Source: Adapted from Senge, 1990.

Although called a health care system, our current approach to care is disease-focused "rescue medicine," which is extremely expensive and contributes to the symptom of increased cost.

As Figure 11.2 shows, there are two alternatives to dealing with this problem: (1) recognize that our disease-oriented approach to care is the fundamental problem and move toward increased emphasis on quality of life through prevention, as well as appropriate palliation; or (2) respond to the symptom of escalating cost with control through commercialization, becoming businesslike to the exclusion of appropriate clinical and ethical considerations.

While the fundamental solution may be more expensive initially and take time to produce the desired results, the symptomatic solution will produce only temporary improvement and disastrous long-term consequences. Providing care in the same way but lowering cost by not giving patients all they need will decrease the quality of care. Over time, costs will rebound because poor quality is ultimately more expensive, due to the cost of complications, complaints, and poor outcomes. The response to increased costs

Figure 11.2. Health Care Costs, Quality, and Access.

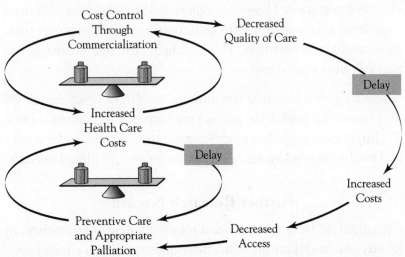

may be decreased access, through implicit or explicit rationing. In an environment of highly restricted access, the transition to more prevention and health-promotion would be even more difficult to accomplish. If an enterprise can't afford transplants, it will surely imagine that it can't afford mammograms and prenatal care.

Not all forms of prevention save money. For example, early detection of many diseases, such as HIV infection and high cholesterol, may actually result in higher medical costs (Rosenthal, 1997). However, primary prevention interventions, such as prenatal care, have been shown to save as much as $3.38 for every dollar spent (Winslow, 1992). At the other end of the life span, one study found that 13 percent of hospital patients, many of whom were terminal, accounted for more than 50 percent of the costs (Lamm, 1989). I am not advocating assisted suicide but rather a movement toward making treatment decisions based on the likelihood of desirable outcomes suggested by available research, coupled with improvements in the management of dying patients to eliminate needless pain and stress ("Let gravely ill die with dignity," 1997).

My main point is that prevention can work, but the payback is likely to be long-term and community-based. Population-based efforts and chronic illness management are key opportunities for clinical integration. However, organized delivery systems will need long-term relationships with patients in order to recoup their investment in prevention. This highlights the significance of the portable insurance issue.

These themes summarize the authors' wealth of practical advice and lessons for practicing physicians, nurses, and administrators. Yet integration is really a macro-organizational issue, and the next and final section addresses implications for organizational research.

Further Research Needed

Organized delivery systems are a relatively new phenomenon in health care, and there are many more questions about clinical integration than answers:

1. Does clinical integration improve individual patient outcomes?

2. Is there an aggregate effect at the community level?

3. Which mechanisms lead to clinical integration?

4. Which approaches to implementing these mechanisms are most successful?

Such fundamental gaps in our knowledge underscore the need for ongoing systematic evaluation of the outcomes of clinical integration, the effects of suggested mechanisms on integration, and the processes used to implement these mechanisms.

As Shortell, Gillies, Anderson, Erickson, and Mitchell have noted (1996), evaluating the effects of clinical integration requires measurement of variables such as the total cost of care per episode of illness, clinical outcomes, functional health status, patient satisfaction, and, ultimately, the health status of the community served. These researchers also identified barriers that must be overcome to conduct such research, including a lack of appropriate measurement tools and the need for study designs that can isolate the effects of clinical integration from other determinants of community health.

One way to increase our understanding of clinical integration and its relationship to other factors would be to develop a measure of clinical integration that assesses patient and family perceptions of how well their care is coordinated across services and sites within a system. Because patients and their families are the only ones experiencing the care received across the system, their perceptions should be an important indicator of the extent to which information systems, clinical paths, case management, and other mechanisms have achieved the intended goal of clinical integration. Items would address what patients and families in a clinically integrated system could be expected to experience:

1. How often do you have to repeat your medical history during one episode of illness?

2. How familiar are caregivers in one facility with the care you received at another site during an illness?

3. If you have been discharged from a hospital, how often does someone from the health system contact you during your recovery?

The dependent variables of interest could be major clinical outcomes. These variables can be measured for a homogeneous group of patients using the approach to evaluating outcomes as key indicators in a clinical path variance system, as Robertson described in Chapter Eight. After controlling for intensity by entering a set of individual variables (such as age or comorbidities) in the first step of a hierarchical regression analysis, the clinical integration score could be entered in step two to assess its unique contribution to explaining variance in outcome achievement (Keppel and Zedeck, 1989). If the sample of patients was drawn from different systems, which may be desirable to increase variability, a system variable could be entered as step three to determine whether site explains additional variance in outcomes over and above individual patient differences and clinical integration (Rothstein, Borenstein, Cohen, and Pollack, 1990).

This approach could potentially be broadened from a case-type to community level of analysis by collecting data from a random sample of residents from a community that is widely served by an IDS. In this case, the dependent variables would be indicators of community health expected to be affected by clinical integration within the IDS, such as immunization and smoking rates and availability for work or school. Variables describing the community (such as income and education level) would be entered in step one, and the clinical integration score would again be entered in step two to evaluate its unique contribution to community health over and above the demographic variables. Clearly, two key factors that could also influence a system's ability to improve community health status are the percentage of residents enrolled and the length of enrollment. Consideration would have to be given to these factors in selecting communities to study.

Although this type of cross-sectional, correlational research would not provide evidence of causation (that is, that clinical integration causes a better outcome), it may contribute to our understanding of relationships between clinical integration and other variables. Findings from systematic study of clinical integration and its outcomes and antecedents will be critical to the organization of health care delivery in the coming years.

Conclusion

For an industry that has been doing "business as usual" for decades, health care organizations are making remarkable changes. Early signs suggest the day may be coming when *health care system* will no longer be a misnomer in this country. This book should assist emerging delivery systems in their progress toward that goal.

References

Keppel, G., & Zedeck, S. (1989). *Data analysis for research designs*. New York: W. H. Freeman.

Lamm, R. D. (1989, August 2). Saving a few, sacrificing many—at great cost. *The New York Times*.

Let gravely ill die with dignity. *Hospitals and Health Networks, 71*(13), 52.

Rosenthal, E. (1997, March 16). When healthier isn't cheaper. *The New York Times*, section 4, p. 1.

Rothstein, H. R., Borenstein, M., Cohen, J., & Pollack, S. (1990). Statistical power analysis for multiple regression/correlation: A computer program. *Education and Psychological Measurement, 50*, 819–830.

Senge, P. M. 1990. *The fifth discipline: The art and practice of the learning organization*. New York: Doubleday.

Shortell, S., Gillies, R. B., Anderson, D. A., Erickson, K. M., & Mitchell, J. B. (1996). *Remaking health care in America: Building organized delivery system*. San Francisco: Jossey-Bass.

Ummel, S. L. (1997). Pursuing the elusive ID. *Healthcare Forum Journal, 40*, 73–76.

Winslow, R. (1992, May 1). Infant health problems cost business billions. *The Wall Street Journal*, p. B1.

Index